A Concise Guide to the Mental Capacity Act

This book provides a clear introduction to the Mental Capacity Act (MCA, 2005), offering an easy reference guide to the complex issues enshrined within the Act to inform the everyday practice of those who need to perform within its parameters as part of their day-to-day work.

Bringing together clinical neuropsychology expertise with legal commentary, the book introduces the main principles and presumptions of the MCA (2005) and describes the processes involved in the comprehensive assessment of what can, in practice, be complex issues. It provides learning summaries, flowcharts, checklists and web references for easy to access resources. The chapters also contain a broad range of illustrative case examples with considerable emphasis given to those areas of complexity that are not addressed in current guidance and which often prove contentious in everyday practice, such as how particular forms of brain injury can lead to hidden difficulties with decision-making which can be challenging to assess and evidence in practice.

The book is essential reading for trainee nurses, doctors, paramedics, social workers, lawyers, psychologists and health and social care support workers, as well as experienced health and social care professionals such as ward managers and care and nursing home managers who face mental capacity issues in their day to day working role.

Dr Tracey Ryan-Morgan is an HCPC Registered Consultant Clinical Neuropsychologist, an Associate Fellow and Chartered Member of the British Psychological Society, as well as a Chartered Scientist and a Regional Fellow of the Royal Society of Medicine and is listed on the Specialist Register of Clinical Neuropsychologists. Tracey consults across the UK and in Harley Street, London.

Understanding how Acquired Brain Injury impacts upon decision making and, therefore, potentially upon Mental Capacity is essential for health and social care staff. This book provides straightforward and structured guidance to aid the process. The use of detailed and multi-layered case studies helps the reader remain grounded in the real world, with all of its complexities and nuances.

— **Dr Mark Holloway**, *Senior Brain Injury Case Manager & Expert Witness*

This book is an essential read for anybody working with people who lack mental capacity and for those professionals tasked with assessing mental capacity. Filled with excellent examples and references to relevant case law, Dr Ryan-Morgan's excellent book covers the basics of the Mental Capacity Act and capacity assessments through to the most complex of issues such as the frontal lobe paradox.

— **Dr Peter Marshall**, *Consultant Neuropsychiatrist*

A Concise Guide to the Mental Capacity Act

Basic Principles in Practice

Dr Tracey Ryan-Morgan

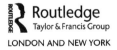

Routledge
Taylor & Francis Group

LONDON AND NEW YORK

First published 2022
by Routledge
2 Park Square, Milton Park, Abingdon, Oxon OX14 4RN

and by Routledge
605 Third Avenue, New York, NY 10158

*Routledge is an imprint of the Taylor & Francis Group,
an informa business*

© 2022 Tracey Ryan-Morgan

British Library Cataloguing-in-Publication Data
A catalogue record for this book is available from the
British Library

Library of Congress Cataloging-in-Publication Data
A catalog record for this book has been requested

ISBN: 978-1-032-07064-3 (hbk)
ISBN: 978-1-032-07059-9 (pbk)
ISBN: 978-1-003-20521-0 (ebk)

DOI: 10.4324/9781003205210

Typeset in Bembo
by Apex CoVantage, LLC

i Simon. *Mi gerddaf gyda thi beth bynnag ddaw.*

Contents

Foreword

You might be forgiven for thinking that capacity law in England and Wales is getting too sophisticated, too juridical, too lawyerish. Are we "assessing" capacity or "determining" capacity? Can someone use and weigh information they do not believe? What is the relevant information for this decision? By the way, what actually is the decision? Is it relating to residence? Or care and support? Or a bit of both? What about "executive functioning" and the frontal lobe paradox? And let us not forget the causative nexus. Do not even get me started on fluctuating capacity. Is this a one-off decision or decision of a continual nature? Is capacity time-specific or should a longitudinal view be taken? Oh, and what about macro and micro decisions?

Then there are best interests. Should we use an objective, subjective or objectively subjective approach? How should we resolve the person's past wishes with their present ones? How do wishes differ from feelings? Or beliefs? And what about values? How much weight should we give to each? Is there a hierarchy? Perhaps we should just ditch all this and focus on supporting people to exercise their legal (as opposed to mental) capacity? And all that is before we even mention the dawn of the liberty protection safeguards replacing the dusk of their procedural counterparts. Yes, you might be forgiven for thinking that capacity law is getting too lawyerish.

At times like these, we crave something simple to rejuvenate the aching muscle of our mind. Well, this concise guide provides just that: a refreshing blast of legal simplicity. Something to take the edge off, to quench the legalistic thirst of health and social care practitioners. With more than 30 practice examples to complement its summary of the law, not to mention checklists, flowcharts, summaries and professional musings galore. Capacity assessors, brain injury service managers, nurses, neurologists, Court of Protection deputies, social workers and occupational therapists all share their thoughts and experiences in an endeavour to bring the law to life.

For let it not be forgotten that the bulk of the Mental Capacity Act 2005 operates outside the Court of Protection, in the nooks and crannies of millions of people's everyday lives. It is a law for the masses, not the preserve of the lawyers. And if the language of the law cannot be translated into everyday life, it serves no useful purpose. It risks becoming inaccessible. Unusable. An irrelevance.

Thankfully, Dr Ryan-Morgan brings her experience of neuropsychology to bear in this easily digestible guide. If the quality of a book is judged by whether its content lives up to the promise of its title, it is a clear success. It is concise, with six chapters. It guides you. It brings the Act back to its basics. And it draws upon a range of specialisms to provide a principled approach to real life practice. In short, it illustrates law put simply. Enjoy.

Neil Allen
Barrister, 39 Essex Chambers

Chapter 1

Introduction to the Mental Capacity Act (2005)

1   What is the Mental Capacity Act (2005)?

The Mental Capacity Act (MCA, 2005) is a piece of statutory legislation which is concerned with balancing the rights of the individual to make decisions with the need to protect those who are vulnerable as a result of impairment to the mind or brain. The Act focuses on the person making a specific decision at a specific time. Any test of capacity is always a legal, and not a clinical, one. The Act only applies to England and Wales and, currently, only to adults.

2   Five principles of the Mental Capacity Act (2005)

i)   A <u>presumption of capacity</u> – every adult has the right to make his or her own decisions and must be assumed to have capacity to do so unless it is proved otherwise. The Vice President of the Court of Protection, Hayden J, stated that:

> There is only one presumption in the MCA, namely that set out at Section 1 (2) i.e. 'a person must be assumed to have capacity unless it is established that he lacks capacity'. This recognition of the importance of human autonomy is the defining principle of the Act. It casts light into every corner of this legislation.[1]

ii) The right for individuals <u>to be supported to make their own decisions</u> – people must be given all appropriate help (and

1 Hayden J [2019] EWCOP 22, paragraph 53, sub-paragraph (h).

DOI: 10.4324/9781003205210-1

information) before anyone concludes that they cannot make their own decisions. The information should be accessible, relevant and tailored to their individual needs, supported wherever possible, practicable and relevant by aids to augment their ability to take it on board (National Institute for Health and Care Excellence, NICE, 2018, paragraph 1.1.5).

iii) Individuals must retain the right to make what might be seen as <u>eccentric or unwise decisions</u>. This is an interesting principle that leads to all kinds of misunderstandings. One needs to seek evidence of the person demonstrating a logical and consistent train of thought. You might ask whether the person is able to evaluate risk and whether they have considered the consequences of action/inaction in arriving at their decision. If the answer is "yes", it may be no more than an unwise decision. If the answer is "no", then there may be grounds to question their mental capacity to make that particular decision. A rule of thumb that may be helpful in your deliberations is to consider when an "unwise" decision could also be classed as an "unsafe" one. At this point, there may be grounds to look closer, using the Mental Capacity Act as a framework. However, there is a note of caution expressed by Jackson J, who had stated that:

> The temptation to base a judgement of a persons capacity upon whether they seem to have made a good or bad decision, and in particular on whether they have accepted or rejected medical advice, is absolutely to be avoided. That would be to put the cart before the horse or, expressed another way, to allow the tail of welfare to wag the dog of capacity. Any tendency in this direction risks infringing the rights of that group of persons who, though vulnerable, are capable of making their own decisions.[2]

iv) <u>Best interests</u> – anything done for or on behalf of people without capacity must be in their best interests (see Section 6 to follow for a definition and for guidance as to the process).

---

2 *Heart of England NHS Foundation Trust v JB* [2014] EWHC 342 (COP), paragraph 7.

v) <u>Least restrictive intervention</u> – anything done for or on behalf of people without capacity should be an option that is least restrictive of their basic rights and freedoms – as long as it is still in their best interests.

Paragraph 1.5.15 of the NICE Guidance (2018) provides some useful pointers (pp. 29–30):

- *What the person would prefer, including their past and present wishes and feelings, based on past conversations, actions, choices, values or known beliefs;*
- *What decision the person who lacks capacity would have made if they were able to do so;*
- *All the different options should be considered;*
- *The restrictions and freedoms associated with each option (including possible human rights infringements); and*
- *The likely risks associated with each option (including the potential negative effects on the person who lacks capacity to make a decision – for example, trauma or disempowerment).*

It should be noted that "*least restrictive*" does not mean <u>non-</u>restrictive. Justice Hayden stated:

The obligation of this Court to protect P is not confirmed to physical, emotional or medical welfare, it extends in all cases and at all times to the protection of P's autonomy.[3]

Key Learning Points	• The Mental Capacity Act is about adults making decisions.
	• There are five principles which underpin the Act.
	• Any assessment of mental capacity must start from a presumption of capacity.

3 What are the key elements of a Mental Capacity assessment?

a) <u>Diagnostic test</u>

> The diagnostic test requires that there is evidence of impairment to the mind or brain which may be temporary or permanent. If this test is not met, there should be no further assessment of mental capacity.

b) <u>Functional test</u>. Here the person being assessed must be able to:

> i **Understand** the "salient facts". The assessor must establish the "Threshold of Understanding" (see Paragraph 5(f)) and assess the person's ability to understand the reasonably foreseeable consequences of reaching a decision or failing to do so, as outlined in s.3(4) of the MCA.

> ii **Recall**. The question is, how long does someone need to remember the information for? How much do they need to remember? "*The person must be able to hold the information in their mind long enough to use it to make an effective decision*" (paragraph 4.20, page 47 of the Code of Practice). However, the assessor should ensure that all assistance is provided in terms of visual aids, written material, prompts, gestures and cues to support a person's ability to recall the information pertinent to the decision.

> iii **Weigh up and use**. Ruck-Keene & Ors (2021) cite a helpful case in describing this aspect of the test as:

>> "*The capacity to actually engage in the decision-making process itself and to be able to see the various parts of the argument and to relate the one to another*".[4] The person only needs to be able to weigh the salient, relevant factors, not all factors, in being able to reach a decision. There is a difference between the person

4 *The PCT v P, AH & the Local Authority* [2009] EW Misc 10 (COP)

being unable and not wishing to give weight to a piece of relevant information.

iv **Communicate the decision once made**.
Once the assessment reaches this limb, it should be clear whether or not the person has capacity to make the decision. This element only refers to the person's ability to communicate the decision, <u>once made</u>. It, therefore, will only refer to a small number of individuals, and, once again, the onus is on the assessor to maximise the person's ability. NICE (2018), in paragraph 1.4.17, page 23, states:

> "*This may include involving an interpreter, speech and language therapist, someone with sensory or specialist communication skills, clinical psychologists or other professionals to support communication*". It might involve the use of communication aids or assistive technology.

c) <u>Causative nexus</u>

What is the causative nexus? Essentially, this refers to the requirement to evidence that the person's impairment of mind or brain is the *reason* why they are unable to make a specific decision at the material time. It is important to be clear that it is not enough for the impairment to make it difficult to make a decision. It has to be the case that <u>because</u> of the impairment, the person is <u>unable</u> to make the material decision.

d) <u>What about decisions that have a different legal test?</u>

The legal test of mental capacity does not have universal application, as there are some decisions in which there are specific legal tests already established that the assessor needs to be aware of. For example:

i **To have sex**. This issue is currently before Supreme Court but, at time of writing, is focused on the capacity to engage in (throughout the act of), rather than consent to (at the start of the act of), sexual relations. Current case law refers to the decision being "issue"- and not "person"-specific. However, the focus on the ability to <u>weigh up</u> the relevant information in arriving at the decision remains key.

ii   **To marry**. The test for capacity here is that the issue is "status"- rather than "person"-specific. The person must understand the broad nature of the marriage contract and also the duties and responsibilities that go with it. The person must not lack capacity to engage in sexual relations.

iii **To make a Will**. This requires the person to have an understanding of what a Will is, of their assets, of who may reasonably expect to benefit at their death and also to be free of any "disorder of mind".

iv   **To make a gift**. The threshold for mental capacity for this action is that the person is capable of *"understanding the effect of the deed when its general purport has been explained to him"*. The degree of understanding is held to be relative to the transaction.

v   **To enter into a contract**. This refers to a specific contract at a particular point in time and not to contracts in general. The person must be capable of understand the nature and effects of the contract that they are proposing to enter into and to be in agreement with them.

vi   **To litigate**. If a lack of capacity is not considered or mitigated in legal proceedings, then the proceedings ultimately can have no effect. What is critical in any assessment of capacity to litigate is the level of understanding required. Case law[5,6] has established that a person might be able to litigate in a simple matter but not a more complex one and must be able to grasp the potential outcomes to proceedings.

e) <u>What about other elements of the MCA?</u>

The issue of Deprivation of Liberty is considered separately and in depth in Chapter 3. However, the Mental Capacity

---

5 [2004] EWHC 2808 (Fam)
6 [2017] EWCOP 5

Act also encompasses other aspects of decision-making that are not commonly referred to. These include:

i   **Capacity to consent to participate in research**. The Act is designed to protect those who may have retained capacity to consent at the outset of a piece of research but lost their capacity to continue to consent as the research progressed. Similarly, the Act covers those who may lack capacity to consent but might, nevertheless, benefit from taking part.

ii   **Capacity to make Advanced Decisions/Living Will**. This is clearly defined in terms of what can and cannot be included (and, therefore, refused at the relevant time). Specifically, a person can make a provision to refuse artificial hydration and nutrition but cannot refuse basic care.

iii **Capacity to make a Lasting Power of Attorney (LPA)**. Many people do not realise that an LPA must be made and registered before the person loses their capacity to make personal decisions. An LPA cannot be sought once capacity is lost.

iv   **The criminal acts of Neglect and Wilful Mistreatment**. The Act makes provision to protect the person lacking capacity from harm by others. Neglect typically refers to a failure to carry out an act that forms part of a duty of care to the patient. Wilful mistreatment is where the act is deliberate or reckless.

v   **Court-Appointed "Deputies"**. These are, typically, Solicitors. Family members may be appointed but this tends to complicate relationships and leads to a blurring of roles and responsibilities that the Court of Protection moves to avoid. Deputies are accountable for all of their actions which are tightly defined and boundaried.

Readers are directed to Ryan-Morgan (2019) for detailed consideration of these elements of the MCA.

Key   An assessment of mental capacity proceeds through
Learning   three key consecutive steps:
Points

1) Diagnostic test. If the threshold is met, then
    proceed to . . . .
2) Function test. If the threshold is met, then
    proceed to . . . .
3) Establish that the person cannot make the decision
    because of the effect of 1 on 2.

Be aware that there are specific legal tests for
certain tests of mental capacity.

4   Who can/should assess a person's mental capacity?

a)   A capacity assessment is, in many ways, an attempt to have
     a real conversation with the person on their own terms
     and applying their own value system. The person assess-
     ing capacity should be someone (carer or professional)
     who knows the person best at the time the decision is
     required to be made. If a specific treatment or examination
     is required, then the professional proposing these should be
     the one carrying out the assessment. Even when there are
     several members of a clinical or care team involved in care,
     it is the person who will be carrying out the intervention
     that is ultimately responsible for the assessment. However,
     a note of caution is sounded where Baker J observed in
     paragraph 16:

> *In assessing the question of capacity, the court must consider all
> the relevant evidence. Clearly, the opinion of an independently
> instructed expert will be likely to be of very considerable im-
> portance, but in many cases the evidence of other clinicians and
> professionals who have experience of treating and working with
> P will be just as important and, in some cases, more import-
> ant. In assessing that evidence, the court must be aware of the
> difficulties which may arise as a result of the close professional*

> *relationship between the clinicians treating and the key professionals working with P.*[7]

It is the case that the more complex the treatment, the more complex the decision. This might mean that the assessment has to be more formal and involve cognitive testing which should only be carried out by someone with the professional training to interpret the results.

The NICE Guidance (2018) exhorts the assessor to build trust with the person being assessed and to take a *"personalised approach"* to the assessment (paragraph 1.2.4).

b) The role of the Court is determinative – the view of the professional who has carried out the assessment may not be. This is because mental capacity is essentially a legal test and not a clinical one. Hayden J points out that:

> *One of the central difficulties faced by practitioners, both in the court setting and in the wider community, is that the relevant tests for capacity are framed by psychologists, psychiatrists etc and a practice has developed of applying these tests as if they had the force of statute. It is necessary to emphasise that when an application is made to a judge, it is the judge who evaluates the broad canvas of evidence to determine the question of capacity. In simple terms, it is judge not experts who decide these issues.*[8]

Key Learning Points	• An assessment of mental capacity should be thought of as a conversation with the person.
	• It should be carried out by someone who knows the person well or, if more complex, by the appropriate professional.
	• The assessment should be individually tailored.
	• Mental Capacity is, ultimately, a legal test which is for the Courts to decide upon.

7 *PH v A Local Authority* [2011] EWHC 1704
8 [2019] EWCOP 27, paragraphs 42 & 43

5   How should the assessment be approached?

a)   <u>According to NICE 2018, an effective assessment</u> is:

> *Thorough, proportionate to the complexity, importance and urgency of the decision, and performed in the context of a trusting and collaborative relationship* (p. 12).

b)   <u>*It is important to remember that P has to 'prove' nothing. The burden of proving a lack of capacity to take a specific decision always lies upon the person who considers that it may be necessary to take a decision on their behalf (or will invite a court to take such a decision). The standard of proof which must be achieved is on the balance of probabilities. . . . Accordingly, it will always be for the decision maker to prove that it is more likely than not that P lacks capacity*</u> (Ruck-Keene & Ors, 2021, paragraph 8, pages 2–3).

c)   <u>You must be clear that there are reasonable grounds for carrying out the assessment.</u> Ruck-Keene & Ors (2021, paragraph 13, page 4) cite an example of a case in which the Court of Protection decided that it was not necessary or appropriate to order a further capacity assessment in a case in which (1) nothing was actually going to turn on the outcome of that assessment and (2) the very process of carrying out that assessment might itself cause P anxiety and distress.[9] The point is that the assessment itself can be seen as intrusive by the person, who may refuse to participate or co-operate.

d)   <u>The assessor must set the "*threshold of understanding*" prior to commencing the assessment.</u> Case law has established that the person being assessed needs only to understand the "*salient factors*".[10] The judiciary has also been clear to assessors that the bar must not be set too high.[11] Finally, assessors are reminded that the person should not be treated as a "*blank canvas*" as professionals may attach too much weight to their own views regarding the person and how to protect them.[12]

---

9   *Re SB (capacity assessment)* [2020] EWCOP 43
10   *LBJ v RYJ* [2010] EWHC 2664 (Fam).
11   *PH and a Local Authority v Z Limited & R* [2011] EWHC 1704 (Fam).
12   *CC v KK & STCC* [2012] EWHC 2136 (COP).

e) The Code of Practice guidance makes it clear that the assessor must provide maximum support to the person being assessed and that this might require multiple visits (paragraph 3.14).

NICE (2018) guidance gives clear direction as to how to provide information to the person being assessed in that it should be accessible, relevant and tailored to their specific needs (paragraph 1.1.5) and that assessors should recognise the best time to make the decision, provide information about the consequences of making or not making the decision and should know what importance the person might attach to key considerations involved in making the decision (paragraph 1.4.8).

f) The assessor must be careful not to conflate their assessment and conclusion. Ruck-Keene & Ors (2021, paragraph 5) state that, in their experience, the word "*assessment is . . . all too often used to cover two completely different things: (1) the process of assessing . . . and (2) the recording of the conclusion*".

In essence, the assessor needs to show their workings. This has been earlier advised by NICE (2018) in which the assessor is guided to record:

- *What the person is being asked to decide;*
- *How the person wishes to be supported to make the decision;*
- *Steps taken to help the person make the decision;*
- *Other people involved in supporting the decision;*
- *Information given to the person;*
- *Key considerations for the person in making the decision;*
- *Whether on the balance of probabilities a person lacks capacity to make a decision;*
- *The person's expressed preference and the decision reached;*
- *Needs identified as a result of the decision;*
- *Any further actions arising from the decision; and*
- *Any actions not applied and the reasons why not* (paragraph 1.2.17).

g) What about when the person appears to have fluctuating capacity?

Fluctuation can be over a period of hours, days, weeks or even longer and is very much an individual consideration for the assessor. In this context, Ruck-Keene & Ors (2021, section D) differentiate between whether a decision is a one-off or represents repeated decisions. A one-off decision may be able to be delayed until the person is likely to re-gain capacity, although this does depend on the nature of the decision. Repeated decisions, also referred to as "*performative*" (see Chapter 5, Cameron & Coddling, private correspondence, for further consideration of this concept) require a series of micro (and connected) decisions. In such cases, the assessor must take a broader view such that if there are only brief periods during which the individual can make capacitous decisions, the conclusion must be that they lack capacity.

Examples of fluctuating capacity are cited in[13] relation to a person's ability to manage their diabetes and in a separate case[14] which relates to a woman's lack of capacity to make decisions about birth arrangements.

However, a note of caution was sounded by Newton J in the comment:

> *The interrelationship between the micro and macro-decisions still needs to be decided, having regard to a particular individual in particular circumstances and having regard to their particular condition. No two people self-evidently are ever the same, their condition the same condition, or the circumstances the same.*[15]

This issue had been previously considered by the Court of Appeal, "*where a decision is of a kind which falls to be made on a daily or at any rate repeated basis, it is inevitable that the inquiry required by the Act is as to the capacity to make a decision of that kind, not as to the capacity to make any particular decision of that kind which it may be forecast may confront the protected person.*"[16]

13 *RB Greenwich v CDM* [2018] EWCOP 15
14 *United Lincolnshire Hospital NHS trust v CD* [2019] EWCOP 24
15 [2019] EWCOP 32, paragraph 47
16 [2014] EWCA Civ 37, paragraph 84

h) <u>The assessor has a responsibility to inform the person as to the support available through advocacy</u> (paragraph 1.1.7, NICE, 2018), including:

- *Enabling them to make their own key decisions; and*
- *Facilitating their involvement in decisions that may be made . . . under the Mental Capacity Act.*

i) <u>What do you do if the person refuses to co-operate with the assessment?</u>
Ruck-Keen & Ors (2021, section F), seek to differentiate between those who are unwilling and those who are unable to take part in decision-making. If unwilling, the Code of Practice (paragraphs 4.57–4.59) suggest explaining the reasons for the assessment and the potential consequences of not participating. If the person is unable to agree or refuses to participate, the assessment can go ahead and the Best Interests route needs to be followed.

Cobb J considered what conclusions can be drawn when a person refuses, deliberately, to co-operate with a capacity assessment:

> *It seems to me that the patient's lack of engagement or cooperation with the assessment may contribute in itself to a conclusion that a patient is unable to understand the information relevant to the decision . . . and/or (perhaps more significantly, if the patient is shown to understand) unable to use or weigh that information as part of the process.*[17]

Key Learning Points	When assessing mental capacity, the assessment should be:
	• Thorough,
	• Balanced,

17 *Re P* [2014] EWHC 119 (COP)[2] www.bailii.org/ew/cases/EWCOP/2017/36.html

- Have a clear justification,
- Be set at an appropriate level of expectation of the person,
- Be supportive to the person,
- Be transparent in terms of process and conclusion,
- Take into account any fluctuations of capacity, and
- Be respectful of the person's wishes.

Case example 1: capacity for property & affairs

Mr **AA** was a 50-year-old gentleman who sustained a traumatic brain injury after falling downstairs at home whilst under the influence of alcohol. He was unconscious at the scene and, when admitted to A&E, was found to have extensive bleeding in his brain requiring emergency neurosurgery to remove large clots.

As the months went by and he remained in hospital receiving active neurorehabilitation, he was observed to have limited awareness of his injury or its impact. His speech was convoluted and verbose. He remained confused and chronically disorientated with significant gaps in his autobiographical memory, such as remembering where he lived. As this all occurred during the COVID-19 pandemic, there was no visiting at the hospital and contact with family was by telephone. His wife was difficult to contact and rarely answered her phone or attended scheduled (virtual) meetings with the clinical team.

It became clear that prior to the injury, **AA** and his wife had been about to separate. He had no recollection of this. During his hospital stay, he was approaching the age at which his occupational pension was about to become accessible, and concerns were raised about his ability to make decisions around such a large sum of money, particularly as he may have been about to enter divorce proceedings. He had begun to express concerns about his wife spending their joint monies on large purchases (such as new car) without reference to his wishes.

Assessment flowchart with worked examples

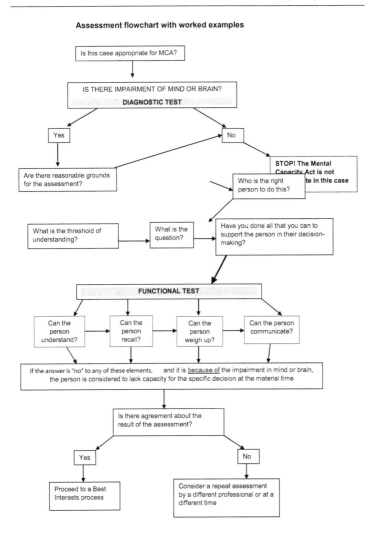

An early assessment of his financial awareness had confirmed his lack of mental capacity to make decisions regarding his finances, particularly as he was disorientated and unable to recall any information about his bank accounts or income.

As the months progressed, he continued to make improvements in cognitive function and ability, and a re-assessment of his ability to manage his property and affairs was indicated.

During the interview, he was orientated but remained verbose and distractible, and it was extremely difficult for him to maintain topic without significant prompting and direction. Cognitive testing indicated that he was functioning at or around the 25th centile (low average) but that he was still unable to consider financial information in context and in relation to financial commitments (weighing up). He continued to be confused about income sources or amounts. Although this could be rectified by obtaining, and providing him with, that information, his continued inability to use information to arrive at financial decisions pointed to the conclusion that he continued to lack mental capacity to manage his property and affairs. This would be the case whether or not he and his wife reconciled or proceeded with divorce. He was asked whether he wanted any information about his finances, to support any decision-making or inform a Best Interests approach, and he declined. He was, thereafter, considered a Protected Party. As he was still in recovery and participating in active neurorehabilitation, the situation would continue to be reviewed at appropriate intervals.

This case demonstrates the importance of keeping matters under review and of re-assessing when there has been a material change in a person's circumstances.

Case example 2: capacity to decide discharge destination

Mrs **AB** was a 55-year-old woman who was diagnosed with limbic encephalitis. This is a condition in which the body releases antibodies against itself and the brain becomes inflamed. She presented with fluctuating confusion and disorientation several months post-diagnosis. Her brain scans pointed to permanent changes throughout her cortex (white brain matter).

AB lived alone prior to her illness and was fully independent. She had close family nearby and many friends in the local community, where she had lived all of her life.

Following a period of intensive neurorehabilitation, she did become more orientated and slowly recovered more autobiographical information relating to her pre-illness working and family life, including the fact that she had been a local taxi driver for many years. Her awareness of the impact of her brain pathology also developed to the point where she knew that her memory *"was not right"*. However, she was keen to return home and to work. Her behaviours on the ward and during assessment led to concerns being raised about the mismatch between the level of support and prompting she required in order to function in a structured ward environment and the fact that she lived alone and would need to be able to identify and manage her own needs on a daily basis in order to be discharged home.

Formal cognitive testing provided objective evidence of **AB** experiencing significant difficulties with attention and concentration, getting new information into memory (new learning), processing speed as well as with visuospatial skills (visual field difficulties). When the results were discussed with her, **AB** made light of them, stating that she had, *"never been very good at school"*. Standardised testing always compares the person to how they would have performed pre–brain injury and/or against age peers.

Time was spent with **AB** exploring what she might need when discharged home, and she responded well with guided insight. The process was closely supported by her family, one of whom planned to move in with her temporarily to provide assistance and prompting.

A pre-discharge home trial was set up, initially just for a few hours in the day, eventually reaching an overnight stay. As the trial progressed, any difficulties were responded to by the clinical team on the ward and the family working together.

At this stage, an assessment of **AB**'s capacity to decide her discharge destination was undertaken. By this time, she had personal experience of what would be involved and what her needs might be, as well as more practical information on issue such as how she would obtain a repeat prescription of her medications. With appropriate prompting and guidance, **AB** was able to understand the information relevant to discharge and to retain sufficient information of this for the purposes of the assessment. With support, she was able to weigh up and consider the risks, knowing that there was an informal but fixed care provision from her close family and friends. She had no difficulty in communicating her wish to return home.

This case demonstrates that, despite widespread and significant brain pathology and its effects on cognitive function, it was possible to support **AB** to the point where she demonstrated clearly that she retained the mental capacity to make an informed decision about returning home from hospital.

6   What happens if the person lacks capacity for a decision?

a)   How and when to have difficult conversations about loss of autonomy?

At the point at which it is determined that the person lacks capacity to make a specific decision and it is clear that the next step is to consider their Best Interests, it is essential that they are informed of this. The person sharing this information should be mindful of how to feedback to the person sensitively and reassuringly. You should be prepared to explain how the person who has been deemed to lack capacity has a key role in the subsequent Best Interests process. Consider who should be present to support the person to receive this feedback. Consider providing feedback in the format best suited to the person so that they do not have to rely on a (probably faulty) memory of the conversation. Be prepared to answer questions and to prepare the person for the consultation process which will follow.

b)   Best Interests – what it is and what it is not

The concept of Best Interests is often improperly described and defined by those seeking to establish it for the person deemed to lack capacity. Unfortunately, it is not described in any detail in the Mental Capacity Act (2005), but there is a substantial body of judicial opinion that it is helpful to refer to.

Best Interests is not what the person would have decided for themselves if they were well enough to do so (also called "substituted judgement").

I have deliberately not tried to set out how convinced the court has to be about what P would have decided if he or she was able to do so because, in my view, the weighing exercise is so case and issue sensitive and is not a linear or binary exercise. . . . P's history may show that he or she has made a series of damaging . . . decisions and so although if they had capacity they would be likely to do so again, the court . . . can conclude that it would not be in their best interests for such a decision to be made on their behalf.[18]

Best Interests does not *"say that P's wishes are to be paramount, nor does it lay down any express presumption in favour of implementing them if they can be ascertained".*[19]

c) How do we determine what is in someone's Best Interests? Best Interests is not a decision but a **process** that needs to be transparently and systematically followed in order to arrive at a meaningful conclusion for the person and a course of action that is "least restrictive" of their rights and freedoms as well as balancing their social and emotional welfare alongside their clinical needs, Ruck-Keene & Ors (2020).

Baker J makes it clear that:

There is no theoretical limit to the weight (or lack of weight) that should be given to the person's wishes and feelings, beliefs and values.[20]

Who is the Decision-Maker? The answer to this lies in considering who will be carrying out or implementing the final decision that is made. Ultimately, the decision-maker is accountable for the actions that they take. (In the case of a Best Interests decision for life sustaining treatment, there is established case law to consider, and the decision-maker may have to pursue the matter through the courts if there is no consensus between the relevant parties).

It is important to be clear that a person identified as "next of kin" has no legal authority to make a decision on someone else's behalf.

In following a Best Interests process, the following checklist may be helpful to the decision-maker:

18 [2016] EWCOP 53
19 [2010] 1 WLR 1082 paragraphs 56 & 60
20 [2017] EWCOP 15 paragraph 56

Have you established whether there is a Lasting Power of Attorney, Court Appointed Deputy or Advanced Decision in place?	√/X
Have you clearly documented the decision that needs to be made?	√/X
Have you identified all of the relevant information and circumstances? (What might the person take into account if making the decision for themselves?)	√/X
Have you encouraged the person to participate?	√/X
Have you established the person's past and present wishes and feelings, beliefs and values? (These may have been expressed verbally in writing, in behaviour or habit – see Code of Practice p. 65.)	√/X
Can you be sure that you have avoided discriminating against the person?	√/X
Have you consulted those people important to the person? (Be mindful of the person's right to confidentiality.)	√/X
Have you established the person's rights (and respected these)?	√/X
Have you clearly documented all of the processes you have followed?	√/X
Have you identified clear options for the person as a result of following the Best Interests process?	√/X
For each option, have you clearly identified the risks and benefits as well as the likelihood of each occurring so that weight can be given to each in terms of identifying restrictions and freedoms?	√/X
Have you clearly documented your considerations of how any risks or disadvantages could be reduced or mitigated in line with a least restrictive imperative?	√/X

Key	•	Prepare the person for the Best Interests process.
Learning	•	Be clear in your own mind about what Best
Points		Interests is and is not.
	•	Follow the process clearly and transparently, being aware that the decision-maker is accountable.
	•	Be careful to avoid discrimination against the person.
	•	Do not be risk-averse in your deliberations.
	•	Consider each decision in its own individual circumstances.
	•	Ensure that your final decision follows the principle of being "*least restrictive*" to the person.
	•	Monitor the situation and if there is material change, consider a review of the decision.

In following this "*balance sheet approach*" (King et al, 2020), be clear why the option you have identified is in the person's Best Interests but do not be tempted to follow a numerical approach in favour of a qualitative one in your determinations.[21]

If there is a dispute or it is not possible to arrive at a consensus, through further meetings or mediation, then the only course of action is to apply to the Court of Protection for a determination of the person's Best Interests.

Those following this process should be mindful that the Court of Protection:

> *Is gradually and increasingly understanding its responsibility to draw back from a risk averse instinct to protect P and to*

21 [2015] EWCOP 76 paragraph 52

> *keep sight of the fundamental responsibility to empower P and to promote his or her autonomy*[22] (Hayden, J).

In following this imperative, it is important to monitor the person's circumstances to see if there has been any material change. If so, the decision in question may need to be reviewed and a new assessment of mental capacity undertaken (NICE, paragraph 1.5.17). For example, the person may achieve an improvement in their cognitive abilities such that their decision-making capacity may no longer be questioned. There is also the possibility that they may experience a reconciliation (or estrangement) in a close relationship which may impact their Best Interests.

References/weblinks

Decision-Making and Mental Capacity. (2018) NICE. www.nice.org.uk/guidance/ng108

King, C.; Coggon, J.; Dunn, M. & Ruck-Keene, A. (2020) An aide-memoire for a balancing act? Critiquing the "balance sheet" approach to best interests decision-making. *Medical Law Review*, 28 (4), pp. 753–780.

Mental Capacity Act Code of Practice. (2007) www.gov.uk/government/publications/mental-capacity-act-code-of-practice

Mental Capacity: Supporting Decision Making after Brain Injury. (2016) Headway. www.headway.org.uk/media/4108/mental-capacity-supporting-decision-making-after-brain-injury-e-booklet.pdf

Ruck-Keene & Ors. (2021) 39 Essex Chambers: Carrying out and recording capacity assessments. https://1f2ca7mxjow42e65q49871m1-wpengine.netdna-ssl.com/wp-content/uploads/2020/12/Mental-Capacity-Guidance-Note-Capacity-Assessment-January-2021.pdf

Ruck-Keene & Ors. (2020) 39 Essex Chambers: Determining and recording best interests. https://1f2ca7mxjow42e65q49871m1-wpengine.netdna-ssl.com/wp-content/uploads/2020/07/Mental-Capacity-Guidance-Note-Best-Interests-July-2020.pdf

Ryan-Morgan, T. (2019) *Mental capacity casebook: Clinical assessment and legal commentary*. Abingdon, UK: Routledge.

22 EWCOP 22 [2019] paragraph 51

Chapter 2

How do we make decisions and how do we assess decision-making?

1   How do we make decisions?

The ability to choose options that lead to advantageous outcomes is important in an individual's social life, individual health management, financial management and profession. However, difficulty making advantageous decisions has been reported both in neurologically healthy individuals and those with psychiatric and/ or neurological impairments, leading to substantial limitations on successful and independent living (Schiebener & Brand, 2015, p. 171).

We make decisions by considering the possible solutions to the problem or the outcomes we wish to achieve after the decision is made. In doing so, one considers previous experiences of decision-making, both in general and also in particular connection to the issue under decision. We may take advice from others or read up on a subject to be better informed. The decision-maker may weigh up the pros and cons or even take their time and postpone the decision until they are "sure" or until it "feels right". Part of this process often involves working out how we will tell others once the decision is made. The steps in the process of decision-making are summarised in the following flowchart:

DOI: 10.4324/9781003205210-2

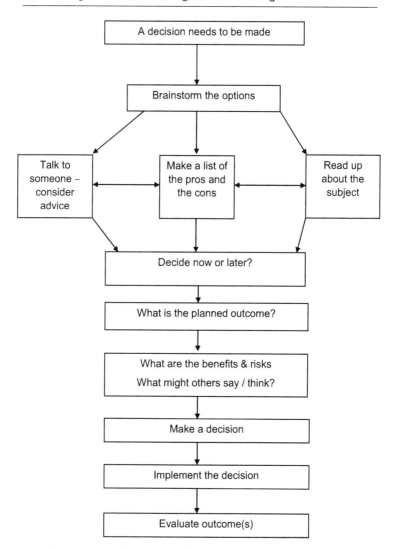

2   Which bits of the brain help us to make decisions?

It is important to understand how decisions are made by the brain. In the healthy brain, there are essentially two competing systems that are activated when we enter into decision-making. The first is referred to as the "impulsive system" and is mediated

Key   •   Decision-making is key to an individual's
Learning   independence and self-expression.
Points   •   Decision-making is a key part of everyday life.
       •   Making decisions forms a complex process of
           formulating, evaluating and implementing our
           beliefs and emotional responses to everyday
           situations.

by a part of the front of the brain called the Orbitofrontal cortex. The second is called the "reflective system" and is underpinned by the Dorsolateral prefrontal cortex. The two systems are moderated by the functions of the Ventromedial prefrontal cortex[1]

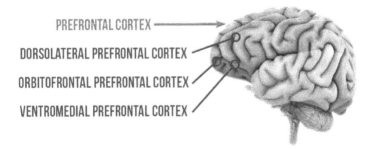

PREFRONTAL CORTEX
DORSOLATERAL PREFRONTAL CORTEX
ORBITOFRONTAL PREFRONTAL CORTEX
VENTROMEDIAL PREFRONTAL CORTEX

The impulsive system is one in which emotional reactions are in the ascendancy. We refer to these as "gut feelings" or "intuition" when we are driven by excitement or the prospect of a reward. The reflective system is where we pause, reason out possible outcomes, plan strategies and think about times where we have made similar decisions in the past, including evaluating what we learned from those moments. The

1 Image taken from: www.google.com/url?sa=i&url=https%3A%2F%2Fwww.thescience ofpsychotherapy.com%2Fprefrontal-cortex%2F&psig=AOvVaw2Q8CrJFAB-biSVS9NYvCGBs&ust=1617023353509000&source=images&cd=vfe&ved=-0CAMQjB1qFwoTCPiXytOH0-8CFQAAAAAdAAAAABAD

ventromedial prefrontal cortex mediates these two systems, analysing risk to the person. It is involved in triggering which system takes the lead. Our whole executive (front of brain) system is important for integrating all of the information from these decision-processes and for developing an overall strategy based on the outcome. Which mode or system takes the lead depends on both the individual and the environment or circumstances of the decision. For example, buying those new shoes that we cannot really afford or having that second piece of chocolate cake is more likely to be mediated by the impulsive system whereas purchasing a new house or considering a new career is more likely to be underpinned by the reflective system.

The individual attributes of the person come into sharp focus in decision-making. Some people are calm when making decisions in a stressful situation, whereas others tend towards impulsive decision-making styles whatever the circumstance. We are all different, but there are factors which influence how we make decisions. For example, a person's age and intelligence play a part but so do their cognitive abilities, executive functions (particularly the ability to inhibit an automatic response) and emotional regulation strategies (Liebherr et al., 2017).

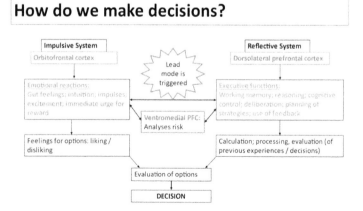

How do we make decisions?

Key   •   The front of our brain is the centre of our
Learning   decision-making processes.
Points   •   There are two competing brain systems in making
                      a decision: the emotional one and the reasoned
                      one.
                 •   Which system takes the lead depends on the
                      person, their values, beliefs and priorities, but it
                      also depends on the environment in which the
                      decision was made, the person's age and their
                      cognitive abilities.

3   How do we assess someone's decision-making abilities when these are in question?

a)   Clinical observations: it is important not to underestimate the power and importance of clinical observation in assessment. Does the person require support or prompting in everyday decision-making? For example, do they choose their own clothes or what and when they eat, when they do their laundry or when they change their bed? Do they choose when to go shopping or how much to spend on a pair of shoes? Can they initiate decision-making by recruiting the information that they already have in order to approach the decision? If a person requires reminding or prompting, then there may be memory issues. If the person requires support to make a decision, such as only being offered an array of two or three options (*do you want coffee or tea?*) instead of making an "open" decision (*do you want a drink?*), this might mean that they have trouble weighing up information because of cognitive overload which has implications for their ability to make decisions.

b)   Cognitive testing: it is possible to undertake brief general cognitive assessments using measures that are freely available on the internet such as the MOCA (Montreal Cognitive Assessment), the ACE (Addenbrooke's

Cognitive Examination) or ones that have to be purchased such as the BCSE (Brief Cognitive Status Exam). These can usually be administered by a health professional with little or no training in their use, as the instructions for administration and scoring are easy to follow and the scoring gives a number which represents either unimpaired or impaired performance on the test in question.

It is also possible to undertake more specific testing using measures that are designed to assess aspects of decision-making in those adults who are believed or known to be cognitively impaired, such as the (modified) Wisconsin Card Sort (a test of cognitive reasoning that is loaded onto attention and working memory) or one of the many versions of the Tower Test (a test of planning and problem-solving). These latter tests are designed to be administered and interpreted by Clinical or Neuropsychologists who are experienced in their use (tests are explained in more detail in Lezak, 2012, pp. 636 & 375 respectively) and can analyse and interpret types of errors made and patterns of responding in terms of what they mean for the individual's ability to make decisions.

It is critically important to have a robust grasp of the strengths and limitations of commonly used cognitive screening instruments if these are to be employed. For example, you need to know what they do and don't measure as well as being able to interpret what the results actually *mean*. For example, on an ACE (Version 3), a score of 88 and above is considered "*normal*", a score below 83 is interpreted as "*abnormal*" and scores between 83 and 87 are classified as "*inconclusive*". But what does the score number actually *mean*? Lezak (Chapter 6) exhorts us:

i)   Not to read too much into our findings without considering a range of individual factors (such as educational attainment or age, for example);

ii) Not to assume that a low score is equal to impairment (healthy individuals exhibit considerable variability in test performance);

iii) Not to rush to conclusions by ignoring evidence which does not quite fit the suspected diagnosis; and

iv) Not to assume that the person is exerting adequate effort on testing (insufficient effort can be both conscious and unintentional).

It is axiomatic in the field of Clinical and Neuropsychology practice that a person is more than just a sum of their scores on assessment tests. Psychometric data form one small, but significant, part of an overall assessment of an individual's strengths and needs.

d) Ask others – Wood & Bigler (2017) suggest that it is "unwise, even negligent, to form opinions on how test performance is likely to influence everyday behaviour without carefully interviewing those with direct experience of the person's real-world behaviour over a period of time", (p. 93) and that "reliance may need to be placed on observations by family and friends" (p. 97). This can be fraught with difficulties, as some families of those with brain injury can often misinterpret the behaviours of the patient. For example, a common sequel to traumatic brain injury is fatigue, as is emotional blunting. Yet families who are not advised of the organic reason for these difficulties often interpret the person as being "lazy" or "thoughtless". That said, the families can still provide a useful and detailed account of how the brain-injured, or neurologically compromised, person lives their daily life from which the skilled professional can infer areas of difficulty or contradiction, particularly in respect of decision-making. Family members can be best placed to observe and report on the changes that the brain injury has wrought as they knew the person before and can compare their current presentation with their pre-injury self.

e) Ask the person: This seems obvious, but it is surprising how often the person at the centre of the assessment is either overlooked or only involved after all other avenues have been explored. It makes no clinical sense to form an opinion about a person's abilities without asking their views. One caveat is that it is not uncommon for a person with a brain injury or neurological compromise to lack insight into, or awareness of, their cognitive and emotional changes and challenges. But that is the reason why the assessor asks others, carries out direct observations and conducts appropriate (objective) testing as an adjunct to the person's self-view.

A good starting point is to ask the person, "*what do you think that you need help with?*". The person who lacks awareness will likely respond that they do not need any help or will just acknowledge the physical support that they might need to wash or dress, for example. This type of response provides the opportunity to ask deeper questions based on information that is already available such as information from family, or clinical staff, about the actual support and prompting that is needed on a day-to-day basis. It is important to understand that there are two separate constructs at play here – intellectual awareness (knowing the facts) and insight (using those facts in the decision-making process).

Key	•	In order to conduct a thorough assessment of a
Learning		person's decision-making abilities, integration of
Points		the following is essential:

- o   Clinical observations
- o   Cognitive testing
- o   Collateral informants (third-party observations)
- o   The person's own views

4   When we have to assess a person's decision-making abilities – what is a good starting point?

The following might be a useful checklist as it combines best clinical practice with advice from the Code of Practice.

What can/does the person decide now?	
Is the decision urgent?	
Is the decision a one-off (decisional) or part of a process (performative)?	
Have you provided all of the relevant information and in a way that best suits/helps the person? (Does the information cover all potential options open to the person?)	
Have you provided all necessary support to the person? (Have you assessed them at the best time of day for them,	
in the place where they are most comfortable, with support from whomever they feel most comfortable with?)	
Do they understand the consequences of not making a decision?	
Can they put off the decision until circumstances change?	

5   How our decision-making can be affected – case examples to consider

Practitioners should take a personalised approach, accounting for any reasonable adjustments and the wide range of factors that can have an impact on a person's ability to make a decision. (NICE Guidance, 2018, paragraph 1.2.4)

The following case examples are presented to illustrate this particular point.

a.   Mental health (bipolar disorder) and emotional dysregulation (brain injury)

Ms **BA** was a 60-year-old woman transitioning from male. She had a long history of bipolar disorder and had several years previously been administered a catastrophic overdose of prescribed medication in error whilst an inpatient being detained under a section of the Mental Health Act. This lithium toxicity had resulted in several months' care in ITU (Intensive Therapy Unit), multiple organ failure and in permanent changes to her brain functioning (in terms of being able to concentrate, to remember new information and to weigh things up). Her poorly controlled bipolar disorder meant that she struggled to modulate her emotional responses to other people and to day-to-day situations. Her treating medic described her as, *"being very driven, chaotic and impulsive: her manner can become garrulous, vexatious and challenging. She has a history of verbal aggression to staff and family members and can become confrontational in behaviour"* (clinical correspondence).

The assessment started with a detailed review of treatment records (including Medication Administration Record charts), interview with health staff in her placement and contact with family.

During the initial interview with Ms **BA**, she alternated between expressing feelings of anger and switching to tears, frequently sobbing. However, the lability was noted to be short-lived, and she would flip between both in a matter of seconds, indicating a lack of emotional self-regulation or insight. She claimed to have attempted suicide two days prior to the assessment but this was not corroborated by the Registered Manager. Her story was often confused and her account tangential. It was difficult to identify a coherent thread and to check her level of understanding of matters. Her emotional presentation contra-indicated the use of formal testing on any of the several occasions that she was visited. Her family were unable to offer assistance, as they were estranged at the time of the assessment. The Registered Manager of the home described a range of difficulties in supporting and caring for Ms **BA**, who denied any need for support and made frequent (unsubstantiated) allegations about care staff, resulting in many refusing to work with her, thus risking her placement.

Her treating medic was of the opinion that *"she cannot give matters sufficient thought and what thought she gives is distorted by her optimism and faulty reality testing"* (clinical correspondence).

The most important matter for Ms **BA** was that she felt listened to. Her reality was all that she knew, and she wanted help to make sense of this in relation to where she lived and what care she needed to support her. She expressed the view that, in the past, none of those employed to provide care have actually understood her, and that her carers have even been guilty of *"breaching confidentiality and being two-faced"*. She was not able to provide any concrete examples of this, however.

Despite every effort to meet her at her level of functioning, it became clear that her view of the world and her decision-making were both hostage to her emotional dysregulation and that as a result of this, she was frequently placing both herself and others at risk.

An informal agreement was drawn up with the home's Registered Manager and Ms **BA** in which her views would continue to be consistently elicited but that there had to be an acknowledgement that there existed a duty of care to ensure her safety at all times. Sadly, this did not prove to be effective, and the care placement broke down.

This is a case where despite every reasonable adjustment being made to support, listen to, support and encourage the person, their "disorder of mind or brain" has interfered with their decision-making abilities to the point where their well-being (and that of others) was placed at risk.

Mr **BB** was a 40-year-old male who had sustained a traumatic brain injury in a pedestrian versus lorry road traffic collision. He was in post-traumatic amnesia for almost three months, indicating a very severe injury to the brain. His injuries to the brain were widespread and resulted in many cognitive and behavioural changes that his wife struggled to accept and manage. He presented as impulsive, verbally disinhibited, restless and often agitated. He had a lowered frustration tolerance and would be argumentative rather than walk away from a potential conflict. These behaviours were all in stark contrast to his pre-injury self.

Cognitively speaking, Mr **BB** was easily distracted and experienced difficulty following conversation and finding words when communicating. He demonstrated poor problem-solving skills and had difficulty organising his thoughts. He would become fixed on a course of action and frequently put himself at risk by being unable to back down. On a number of occasions, he had come extremely close to assaulting his wife, despite the fact that he loved her dearly.

Clinical work with Mr **BB** focused on improving his self-regulation strategies. Every effort was made to assist him in understanding his brain injury, the effects, how best to work with his residual skills and strengths and what help and support he might need. The rationale was to help him to make the right decision (for him) in the moment where it was needed. In the sessions, he would be able to understand and accept the information. However, he continued to fail to apply the strategies in the moment, despite frequent rehearsal. In essence, he experienced a "strategy application disorder" as a result of his brain injury. He would be able to describe the strategies that he needed to use and he understood why he needed to use them but was unable to recognise when they were required. The consequences were that his marriage broke down, and he spiralled into a deep depression.

Key Learning Points   These cases illustrate that, despite every reasonable adjustment being made to support, to listen to and encourage the person being assessed, their "disorder of mind or brain" has interfered with their decision-making abilities to the point where their well-being was placed at risk.

b   Metabolic disorders (Prader Willi Syndrome) and physical health conditions (pain/fatigue)

Ms **BC** was a 31-year-old female in a residential placement. She had a significant medical history including a primary brain tumour on her pituitary gland and a diagnosis of (acquired) Prader Willi Syndrome. This presents as an individual failing to regulate their oral intake because of an insatiable hunger/thirst and can lead to serious medical complications. In the case of Ms **BC**, she began to gain weight at an alarming rate, reaching 180 kilos (approximately 28 stone) at the time of referral. She had developed Type 2 diabetes and was prescribed a long list of medications for co-morbidities. The referral came as the placement staff were unclear as how best to help Ms **BC** to manage (restrict) her intake which they were seeking to help her to do for health reasons.

Staff had tried the following (all with little or no success):

- Dietetics education, advice and diet sheets;
- Written contract with Ms **BC** with agreed-upon rules about food intake;
- Greater involvement in meal planning, shopping and food preparation;
- Positive reinforcement and use of (non-food) rewards; and
- Reducing the amount of food kept on the premises that she could access.

Ms **BC** had a fiancé who also lived at the placement address (in his own space) and who brought her "treats" of food because for him it represented evidence of affection.

In terms of the MCA, Ms **BC** was not obviously cognitively impaired and was reasonably insightful into the effects of her behaviours. However, consideration was given to the argument that her drive for food was organically mediated and therefore not subject to her control, thus rendering her incapacitated in terms of eating and drinking decisions. This issue has been considered by the Court of Protection[2] where there appeared to be little weight given to the influence of biological drive (impulsive system) over reasoning ability (reflective system) in that judgement.

Ms **BD** was a 70-year-old woman who had sustained a severe traumatic brain injury as a result of a car accident. She had extensive orthopaedic injuries which caused her high levels of pain and affected her mobility to the point where she needed mechanical assistance to transfer and to walk. Ms **BD** experienced such post-injury pain and fatigue that she had to be supported through a strict timetable of limited activity and rest in order to maximise her function. Her cognitive impairments were severe, and although she did not have a reliable yes/no response when communicating, she was able to indicate her views. Whilst Ms **BD** could not initiate communication about her needs, if she was asked in an appropriate way she would respond. For example, if one was to ask, "*do you want a drink?*", Ms **BD** would respond "*no*". However, if a member of staff said to her, "*I have made your favourite tea*", and the drink was placed in front of her, she would initiate drinking it. This enabled her care needs to be met safely and in a way which did not undermine her autonomy.

The key approach with this lady was to ensure that she was not engaged in communication unless fully rested and having received the appropriate pain medication. Time was taken to establish a professional relationship such that her idiosyncratic means of communicating was understood and shared. Interviews were brief and directive. Questions had to be asked in a closed manner and repeated in a different form later in the session to ensure that she was not perseverating in her responses. Over time, it was possible to establish a reliable form of communicating with Ms **BD** and in enabling her to make decisions on day-to-day matters.

Key Learning Points   These cases illustrate that physical health problems can interfere to a significant and disabling degree with decision-making and that sufficient cognizance must be given to such issues in the holistic assessment approach.

c   Medication (failure to comply) and substance misuse

Mr **BE** was a 20-year-old male who had sustained a severe traumatic brain injury when he had been struck (as a cyclist) by a police car engaged in a high-speed pursuit. As a result of his injuries, which led to neuro-surgical intervention for brain bleeding and swelling, he developed post-traumatic epilepsy. Despite being on two separate anti-epileptic drugs (AEDs), Mr **BE** continued to experience regular tonic–clonic seizures, which were always prolonged (*status epilepticus*) and inevitably resulted in an emergency admission to hospital. He was greatly distressed by his seizures. It was established that he was at risk of SUDEP (sudden death due to epilepsy).

Mr **BE** would have only a few minutes' warning that a seizure was imminent and so had little time to act. The clinical team supporting him worked with him to ensure that he took that warning period to let others know that a seizure was coming and to place himself (safely) on the floor to minimise injuries.

As the treating team became more familiar with Mr **BE**, it also emerged that he was smoking cannabis on a daily basis (lowering both the effectiveness of his AEDs and the threshold at which his seizures occurred). He considered that cannabis use was an informed and positive decision for him, one shared by his siblings and parents. He was experiencing significant difficulty in adjusting to life post–brain injury and felt that cannabis helped to keep him calm and measured. He would prioritise his cannabis use over his compliance with AED medication.

From a neurocognitive perspective, it was clear from formal assessment that, as a result of his brain injury, he had significant impairments in the functions that underpin decision-making. His thinking was concrete, binary and not amenable to reason. He was unable to foresee consequences to himself, or others, of any actions he might take and was unable to pause and reflect before acting. For example, after one admission to control his seizures, he decided to discharge himself, and whilst his mother and doctor were considering how best to dissuade him, he jumped out of a first-floor window and ran off. On another occasion, he had gone out one Saturday evening to the local town with a friend who was employed as a support worker. Mr **BE** had got separated from his friend. He had no money on him, had lost his mobile phone and so was unable to call either his friend or his mother to ask for help. He was only found after a search had been put in place in the early hours of the morning.

In relation to both his non-compliance with his AEDs and his daily use of cannabis, several appointment sessions were organised to seek to understand his thinking, to offer him information to consider and to assess whether this resulted in any changes to his behaviours. He was given written and verbal information, supported in accessing resources on-line and encouraged to ask questions of his Neuropsychiatrist at his next appointment, in terms of the effects of cannabis on his AEDs and on his seizure threshold. He continued to deny the (factually correct) information that his cannabis use coupled with non-compliance of AEDs was directly (and indirectly) increasing his seizure frequency and risk of death. This denial was considered to be either as a result of his lack of awareness of the impact of his brain impairments (anosognosia) or his poor coping strategies in coming to terms with his life-changing brain injury. Either way, he was given every support in terms of information and prompting (using electronic reminders as medication prompts). as well as wearing a specialist watch to detect seizures and remotely raise the alarm whilst tracking his location. These were considered to be the least restrictive means of supporting his lack of self-protective decision-making.

Mr **BF** was a 25-year-old man who had a life-threatening brain abscess and who underwent neurosurgical intervention to insert two EVD (extra ventricular devices) and a VP (ventriculo-peritoneal) shunt to drain fluid away from the brain. He had a past medical history of IV drug use, deep vein thrombosis (as a result of injecting heroin) and hepatitis C. There was a realistic concern that, following his neurorehabilitation after brain surgery, he would be at risk of returning to the use of illicit substances. His brain injury had resulted in significant cognitive impairment, particularly in relation to his front of brain decision-making functions. He demonstrated, both on the ward and on formal testing, that he was unable to form and manipulate abstract concepts and was also experiencing substantial memory problems.

As with many patients with a frontal brain injury, he presented as completely plausible in conversation but had been observed throughout his lengthy hospital stay to manifestly fail to translate word into deed. The risk for Mr **BF** was that, even without drugs in his system, he was unable to make informed decisions. It was extremely likely that he would persist with his impulsive (rather than reflective) decision-making style post-discharge. To that end, time was spent with Mr **BF** ensuring that he had sufficient information for the underpinning decisions he would be required to make, such as where he might live, what help he might need and how he might keep himself safe in future. The information was presented verbally, in writing and with pictures and was accompanied by a brief summary of the benefits and risks associated with each of his options for him to refer to when participating in decisions-making.

Key Learning Points   These cases illustrate that sufficient consideration needs to be given to the effects of both prescribed and illicit substances on decision-making when undertaking an assessment. In some cases, even in the absence of *acute* effects of substances or medicines, the *chronic* (or long-term) effects may still hinder decision-making.

d   <u>Coercion and influence</u> (use of money as leverage)

Mr **BG** was a 30-year-old man who had sustained a severe (hypoxic) brain injury as a child after ingesting a controlled drug and experiencing a cardiac arrest. He had been under the Court of Protection for his finances since entering adulthood. He had a relative with whom he had an ambivalent relationship but who had intervened in his friendships across the years and had sought to undermine every clinician who had been involved in his care. It was hypothesised that the motivation of this relative was financial, as **BG** had substantial resources.

When seen on his own, **BG** would state that he felt controlled and bullied into the opinions he expressed in the presence of his relative and that he wanted to be free of the situation. On more than one occasion, he sought help to move to a different geographical area and did not pass on his address to the relative. However, he would subsequently retract his statements and restart the relationship.

In terms of supporting **BG** with his decision-making, the starting point had to be the following:

> "*Supporting decision-making capacity effectively requires a collaborative and trusting relationship between the practitioner and the person. It does not involve trying to persuade or coerce a person into making a particular decision, and must be conducted in a non-discriminatory way*" (Paragraph 1.2, NICE, 2018).

There are times when it may be difficult to discern whether the support of a family member or close friend is supportive or coercive, (Ruck-Keene & Ors, 2021, paragraph 50). It can be difficult to establish what is support and what is "undue influence" and, although this is ultimately for the Court to decide, the assessor must be mindful of the issues.

In **BG**'s case, there was a consistent and unavoidable pattern of control, the motivations for which could only be inferred. One of the difficulties was that **BG** was verbally plausible in conversation and would express views that, although not coherent at face value, would be acknowledged and accepted. A clinician who had assessed his mental capacity on a previous occasion had written:

> " **BG** *has limited insight into his cognitive limitations . . . This insight is further hampered by the inconsistent messages he receives from those in his support system. His lack of insight prevents him from adopting appropriate adaptive strategies to compensate the impact of his brain injury and thus increase his level of functioning that is required for increased independence"* (clinical correspondence).

The starting point for the latest assessment had to be one of active listening. **BG** had developed trust issues because of the insecure attachment he had formed with his relative and their constant undermining of the motives and behaviours of the care and support staff appointed to promote his greater independence. He presented as angry, challenging and closed to discussion. Substantial and patient efforts were made to help him to describe his views and concerns and to seek evidence to support these in a non-judgmental way. All contact with **BG** was carefully documented, as the relative had reported all of those who had previously undertaken capacity assessments to their professional bodies and had also challenged them in the courts. Whilst this may represent an extreme example of the possibility of coercion and undue influence, it is a salutary lesson in following the Code of Practice and professional practice guidelines to the letter.

Key Learning Points   The person assessing capacity for decision-making needs to always be mindful of the possibility of coercion and influence which can only undermine the person's autonomy when they may lean towards a decision which pleases or gains the approbation of the influencer but is not, actually, in the best interests of the person.

e   <u>Language/communication barriers</u>
   Ms **BH** was an Eastern-European national who was
working in the UK when she was hit by a bus whilst crossing the road. She sustained a moderately severe traumatic
brain injury which resulted in neurosurgical intervention
and a prolonged stay in an inpatient neurorehabilitation
unit. After a period of intensive, specialist physiotherapy,
she became largely self-managing in terms of her personal care. Her conversation was fluent, but she frequently
struggled to communicate through the medium of English
as it was her second language.
   A few weeks into her hospital stay, it came to light that
there was a possibility of financial abuse having occurred
whilst she was in intensive care. Her daughter had travelled to the UK, accessed her mother's accommodation
and bank accounts, transferred all of the monies into her
own account and returned to Europe. She had given
notice on the apartment and had put her mother's effects
into storage. **BH** had no awareness of this and was surprised when she discovered what had occurred. **BH**
had a partner, although they lived separately. Her partner reported the daughter to the police, and an investigation determined that the daughter had been following the
(documented) advice of the Intensive Care Consultant,
who had not expected **BH** to survive her injuries. The
partner and daughter hated each other, and what ensued
was a protracted series of counter-accusations regarding
financial abuse of **BH**.
   It became clear that assessing **BH**'s mental capacity to
make financial decisions was essential, particularly as she
had been employed at the time of the accident and was still
in receipt of full pay, had a mobile phone contract which
needed to be honoured and had various other financial
commitments.
   Efforts were made to source a local interpreter so that **BH**
could be assessed in her native language. This was considered
important because there are instances of individuals who are
multi-lingual who, after experiencing a brain injury, find

their abilities in the different languages differentially affected. There was the possibility that her ability to make decisions might be better preserved through her native language, and this had to be supported as an avenue of assessment.

Structured questions were prepared and then translated so that both could be administered and her performance in each language compared with the other. Ultimately, her abilities were equally impaired, as her principal difficulties were not with communication but with weighing up information in relation to decision-making, but that had to be established on the balance of probabilities before approaching the Court of Protection.

Key Learning Points   The importance of communication is often overlooked in assessments of mental capacity. Communication is a complex process that can break down or be interrupted in any point in the chain from hearing speech, remembering, processing and understanding what you have heard to generating your response, finding the right words, putting them in order, thinking about how your response will be received and finding the sounds that you need to make in order to speak.

General learning points:

When assessing a person, it is essential to actively listen, to ensure that the person is at their best (not under the influence of drugs or medicines, not tired or in pain) and that the environment is quiet with few distractions and nobody else is present (unless specifically requested by the person). Pay attention to the non-verbal elements of communication. Use communication aids if needed.

How I approach a mental capacity assessment (Julian Hardwick, Social Worker and Best Interests Assessor)

As a social worker, my pragmatic approach to assessing someone's capacity is always to refer to the five principles as a starting point and direction. It sounds simple, but it is about ensuring you have good preparation.

I have covered many different settings when it comes to assessing capacity, from assessing people within the community, hospital, learning disability services, dementia care units, physical disability services and Neurorehabilitation ward patients with acquired brain injury.

You will need to know the basis for the capacity assessment request, in the context of where the person is currently living. You need to ask why this person is considered to lack mental capacity. What is the mental impairment or condition? Is this a temporary or a fluctuating condition? Assessing individuals with neurological conditions can be quite complex, because of the type of neurological condition, and will always assess jointly with clinical staff needing to return several times to complete my capacity assessment. I will speak to relevant professionals who can advise me more about the condition to understand what the cognitive impairment is and how this would affect the person's ability to make a decision for themselves. I would need to establish whether the decision can be delayed for now or whether it is an urgent decision that requires immediate assessment?

It is important to find out what medication they are on as this can have an impact on how they may respond when communicating, as well as observing their mood behaviour, as both can affect their performance during a capacity assessment. I will also find out when is the best time of day to assess the individual. Is the person more communicative in the morning or after lunch? I will ask questions with the relevant people caring for or treating the person. I am always trying to empower the person by ensuring they are assessed under the best possible conditions as, ultimately, I am trying to support and enable the individual to make their own decisions.

Understanding a person's communication needs is exceptionally important. What are the persons communication needs? Are there communication needs/language barriers, sensory needs? Do you need pictorial communication or support from a Speech and Language Therapist to assist? I will try to establish if the person would feel more at ease and relaxed with their carer/family during and assessment or advocate if they have one. It is important to be self-aware of your own communication style and language. Make sure that you avoid jargon or overly complex words. Is your speech fast or low in volume? Does the individual have hearing or sight difficulties that need to be supported, such as by how you sit near the person? When assessing, ensure that they have the appropriate aids (hearing aids, glasses, communication aids) with them during the capacity assessment. Allow sufficient pauses for the person to respond. Ask open questions, such as "what do you think", "how you feel about this", "what would you do?" This approach allows the person to open and expand on their responses. I will also repeat the questions in a different way if I think that the individual is having difficulty understanding what I have just asked.

When it comes to the functional test, in which the person is required to understand, to retain, to weigh up and use information and to communicate their decisions, I will need to be clear about what options are available. For example, when I am assessing someone's mental capacity for care and treatment, I will need to ensure that I understand what care and treatment this person has, or likely to have, what are the risk and benefits of having this care and treatment, and to check this against their threshold of understanding.

In relation to retaining information, I will present the person with the salient factors (i.e., the information needed to make a decision) with the present options available to them to retain, and check if the person is able to retain this by simple memory recall tests. I will ask if the person understood what was just discussed with them and if they can summarise our discussions.

When considering a person's ability to use information and weigh it up, my approach is to support the individual by helping them to understand the risks and benefits of the decision or of not making a decision.

It is important to be respectful by being aware that as individuals we all have differing social values, cultures, diversity and beliefs, and whether this may be a factor that is influencing the individual's decision-making.

I will also document the person's views, wishes and feelings about their decision during the capacity assessment, as this is relevant in case the outcome is the requirement to act in the person's best interests. This takes into account the least restrictive options in terms of their rights and freedoms by upholding their rights to autonomy and independence.

It is essential to understand and support the communication needs of the person by ensuring all practicable support is made available during their capacity assessment.

When the capacity assessment has completed, my decision is always based on the balance of probabilities and, if necessary, I will revisit the capacity assessment process if there are borderline capacity issues to support the person as best as I can.

<u>Spreading knowledge regarding the impact of acquired brain injury is required for all social workers, in practice and in training</u>.

(Holloway, 2014)

References/weblinks

ACE. www.royalberkshire.nhs.uk/ACE-R%20Cognitive%20Assessment.pdf

BCSE. www.pearsonclinical.co.uk/Psychology/AdultCognitionNeuropsycho logyandLanguage/AdultGeneralAbilities/BCSE/BriefCognitiveStatusExam. aspx

Holloway, M. (2014) How is ABI assessed and responded to in non-specialist settings? Is specialist education required for all social care professionals? *Social Care & Neurodisability, 5* (4), pp. 201–213.

Lezak, M. D.; Howieson, D. B.; Bigler, E. & Tranel, D. (2012) *Neuropsychological Assessment* (fifth edition). Oxford: Oxford University Press.

Liebherr, M.; Schiebern, J.; Averbeck, H. & Brand, M. (2017) Decision making under ambiguity and objective risk in higher age: A review on cognitive and emotional contributions. *Frontiers in Psychology, 8,* pp. 2128–2139.

MOCA. www.mocatest.org/

Norman, A.; Holloway, M.; Odumuyiwa, T.; Kennedy, M.; Forrest, H. & Suffield, F. (2019) Accepting what we do not know: A need to improve professional understanding of brain injury in the UK. *Health & Social Care in the Community, 28,* pp. 2037–2049.

Schiebener, J. & Brand, M. (2015) Decision making under objective risk conditions: A review of cognitive and emotional correlates, strategies, feedback processing and external influences. *Neuropsychological Review, 25,* pp. 171–198.

Understanding People Affected by Brain Injury: Practice Guidance for Social Workers and Social Care Teams (BASW). (2019) www.basw.co.uk/resources/ understanding-people-affected-brain-injury

Wood, R. L. & Bigler, E. (2017) Problems assessing executive dysfunction in neurobehavioural disability. Chapter 7 in T. M. McMillan & R. L. Wood (eds.) *Neurobehavioural disability and social handicap following traumatic brain injury* (Second edition). Abingdon, UK: Routledge.

Chapter 3

What do I need to know about depriving someone of their liberty? (With assistance from Karen Jackson, Consultant Solicitor)

1 What is a DoLS?

Many health, social care and legal professionals will have heard of the term "DoLS", or Deprivation of Liberty Safeguards, but there are a significant number that do not understand what this actually means. It can mean two things: a shorthand for the DoLS authorisation and a deprivation of liberty outside that process.

The DoLS came into force in April 2009, as part of the Mental Capacity Act (2005). The European Court of Human Rights determined that the UK legal system was incompatible with the European Convention on Human Rights (ECHR). Article 5 of the ECHR protects a person's rights to liberty.

Deprivation of Liberty is an act by an authorised person or body to deprive a person of their liberty (by controlling their movements in order to keep them safe from harm. The Supreme Court ruled in a case commonly known as "Cheshire West" that there was an "acid test", namely, that a person was deprived of their liberty if they were subject to continuous supervision and control and were not free to leave.

The DoLS is, therefore, a form of safeguard for people who are restricted in this way and is designed to ensure that:

- The arrangements are in the person's best interests (on the basis that they lack the capacity to keep themselves safe);
- The person is appointed someone to represent them (Relevant Person's Representative);

DOI: 10.4324/9781003205210-3

- The person is automatically given a legal right of appeal over the arrangements (Section 21, Mental Capacity Act) to protect those against being detained when it is not in their best interests; and
- The arrangements are reviewed and are only allowed to stay in place for as long as is absolutely necessary.

The Department of Health is supportive of DoLS as a system because it provides the appropriate checks and balances in terms of the care of the individual deemed to lack capacity to consent to such restrictions (see references).

In order to apply for a DoLS for a named person, there is a set process to follow. The following flowchart summarises the decision process that assists the deliberation.

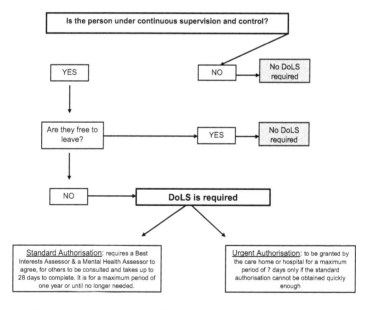

How do you decide if someone is being deprived of their liberty?

The deprivation could be physical, such as on a ward with a keypad entry system or being held by seatbelt in a wheelchair, or it could be pharmacological restraint (such as sedation). It could be the case that the individual is subject to monitoring through sensors or closed-circuit TV systems within the home. It could be that the person can only access the community with support of a member of staff. There might be restrictions on access to food (or to types of food) or prevention of access to alcohol, for example. It might be that there is restricted visiting where the person is accommodated. Although the references are to "continuous supervision and control and not free to leave", it is generally understood that this does not rule out a circumstance in which there are freedoms still amounting to a DoLS restriction. Most importantly for the purpose of deciding whether a plan amounts to a deprivation, a non-capacitous adult's consent or lack of opposition is irrelevant. The person themselves may not agree or may express discontent with the DoLS and can challenge. These are all considerations in the DoLS process.

How can the person subject to DoLS appeal?

Section 21A of the MCA 2005 provides an automatic right of appeal by the person to the Court of Protection. Non-means-tested legal aid is always available to that person to gain legal support in that process.

When a person becomes subject to a DoLS authorisation, there will be two people appointed to support and advise them and to ascertain their wishes and feelings.

The first is an Independent Mental Capacity Advocate, known as an IMCA. Their role is to help the person, P, and the Relevant Person's Representative (RPR) to understand the DoLS authorisation and the relevant rights and how to exercise them and also to help the person or the RPR to apply to court or exercise the right of review.

By contrast with the RPR, it is not the role of the IMCA to work out whether the person would wish to apply to court if they are not able to verbalise or demonstrate this wish or to consider whether there is any other reason to apply to the court to consider the questions in section 21A(2). That is also a matter for the RPR (paragraph 84).

The second is a <u>Relevant Person Representative</u>. The Local Authority must appoint an RPR for every person to whom they give a standard authorisation for deprivation of liberty. This is described as "*a crucial role in the deprivation of liberty process, providing the relevant person with representation and support that is independent of the commissioners and providers of the services they are receiving*".

The RPR must objectively:

- Support the person in matters relating to or connected with the DOLs and
- Take all steps to identify whether they wish to exercise the right to apply to the Court of Protection (or the right to review). If so, it is the RPR's duty to represent and support them in making an application to the Court of Protection, where the RPR concludes that they would wish to make the application in circumstances where they are unable to communicate that wish.

In supporting P, the RPR must assess for himself or herself whether an application should be made to the court in P's best interests, independent of any wishes expressed by P.

The Court of Protection has considered the responsibilities and duties on the IMCA and RPR and the selection of those persons. It has clarified in what circumstances and application should be brought to court on behalf of the person to challenge the authorisation. These two roles can be held by one person if the RPR is a professional appointment, but they can also be held by two separate people if the RPR is a family or friend.

Further information is available on these roles and responsibilities in the judgements provided by Baker J.[1]

A useful flowchart sets out the process:

2   The Process of a DoLS assessment

The person applying for a DoLS authorisation will be what is called the Managing Authority. This will be the manager of

1 [2016] EWCOP 49

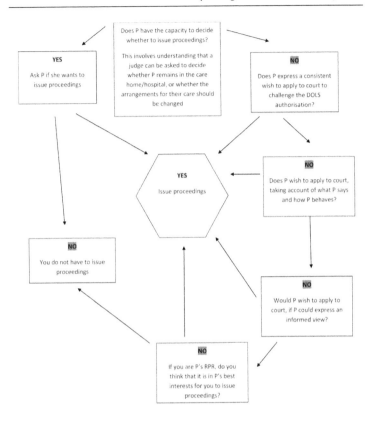

Key Learning Points

- Deprivation of Liberty is a means of restricting a person's freedoms within the terms of the Mental Capacity Act.
- There are specific processes laid down for applying, implementing, monitoring and appealing a DoLS.
- DoLS encompasses many types of restriction to a person.

the residential placement or hospital. An application is made
to the DoLS team who are within the Local Authority. There
are six qualifying requirements that have to be addressed in the
paperwork before authorisation can be granted.

i   The person has to be confirmed as **age 18 or over**
ii There must be **no existing refusal of care or treatment**
    in place (such as an Advanced Decision) or a decision
    already made by an existing Lasting Power of Attorney
    or Court Appointed Deputy (for Health and Welfare
    decisions)
iii An **assessment of mental capacity** of the specific deci-
    sion to be accommodated in the care home or hospital for
    care or treatment
iv A **mental health assessment** (defined by the Mental
    Health Act)
v   An **eligibility Assessment**. This refers to the fact that if
    you are detained under the Mental Health Act, this effec-
    tively "trumps" any consideration for restriction under the
    Mental Capacity Act. This also applies if you are subject
    to a requirement to live in another place (such as by Court
    Order)
vi An **assessment of the person's Best Interests**. This is,
    essentially, an assessment of the proportionality of a DoLS
    in terms of keeping the person safe in the least restrictive
    way. The Best Interests Assessor must take account of the
    views of anyone named by the person as needing to be
    consulted, such as care staff, family, friends, carers and,
    if in place, anyone with a Lasting Power of Attorney or
    acting as a Court Appointed Deputy for the person. If the
    person has no support, then an application can be made
    for an IMCA to provide support.

A Standard Authorisation assessment should not take longer than 21 days to be put in place, but many Local Authorities have very lengthy backlogs. A home or hospital can grant
themselves an Urgent Authorisation, but this can only be
for a maximum of 14 days. Without such authorisation, any

detention is unlawful and may give rise to an unlawful detention claim under the Human Rights Act.

If the conditions are met, then the authorisation is granted, and the person (or their representative) must be given a copy. An RPR must be appointed to represent the interests of the person whose liberty is being restricted. The RPR can be a relative or friend of the person but if they have a conflict (i.e., they think it is in the person's best interests, and the person is in disagreement) then the role will be taken on by a paid RPR who could be the same person as the IMCA.

If there is a change in circumstances of the person during the Standard Authorisation period, then the DoLS has to be reviewed and, if appropriate, removed. A Standard Authorisation can only be granted for a maximum of 12 months. Any longer detention will require a new Standard Authorisation.

There is an automatic right to appeal a DoLS under Section 21A of the MCA. If the person whose liberty is restricted wishes to appeal with the support of their IMCA, or their RPR themselves considers that DoLS is not the least restrictive approach to keeping the person safe, then a challenge can be pursued. This may involve questions being asked about which alternatives were considered and why they were rejected in favour of DoLS.

Key Learning Points

- There are two types of DoLS authorisation: Urgent and Standard.
- DoLS should be considered when there is no lesser level of restriction that would keep the person safe and enable them to receive the appropriate level of care and treatment.
- There are clear processes in place to apply for, implement, monitor, review and appeal a DoLS.

3   Where does an assessment of risk come into consideration?
The purpose of DoLS is to authorise a restrictive care plan by
putting in place a least restrictive option in order to provide
for their health and well-being needs. However, the process of
assessment must weigh up the established risks with the person's right to autonomy and freedom. For example,

> *Physical health and safety can sometimes be bought at too high a
> price in happiness and emotional welfare. The emphasis must be on
> sensible risk appraisal, not striving to avoid all risk, whatever the
> price, but instead seeking a proper balance and being willing to tol-
> erate manageable or acceptable risks as the price appropriately to be
> paid in order to achieve some other good – in particular to achieve
> the vital good of the elderly or vulnerable person's happiness. What
> good is it making someone safer if it merely makes them miserable?*[2]

In the Cheshire West judgement by the Supreme Court,
Lady Hale reiterated this approach in her words:

> *It is axiomatic that people with disabilities, both mental and
> physical, have the same human rights as the rest of the human
> race. . . . (paragraph 45)*
>
> *Those rights include the right to physical liberty, which is guar-
> anteed by article 5 of the European Convention. This is not a
> right to do or to go where one pleases. It is a more focussed right,
> not to be deprived of that physical liberty. But, as it seems to
> me, what it means to be deprived of liberty must be the same for
> everyone, whether or not they have physical or mental disabilities.
> If it would be a deprivation of my liberty to be obliged to live in
> a particular place, subject to constant monitoring and control, only
> allowed out with close supervision, and unable to move away with-
> out permission even if such an opportunity became available, then
> it must also be a deprivation of the liberty of a disabled person.
> The fact that my living arrangements are comfortable, and indeed
> make my life as enjoyable as it could possibly be, should make no
> difference. A gilded cage is still a cage (paragraph 46).*[3]

2 [2007] EWHC 2003 Fam, paragraph 120
3 [2014] UKSC 19

The approach to risk cannot be paternalistic or overly protective. This is a stark reminder of the principle of acting in a way that is in a person's Best Interests **and** is "least restrictive of a person's rights and freedoms". This is usefully referred to by Hayden J:

> *If P lacks capacity, facilitating compliance with a regime to which he is opposed will always involve the lightest possible touch, the minimal level of restraint or restriction and for the shortest period of time.*[4]

The question to ask is, when is a DoLS not a DoLS? Is placing someone under one-to-one support/care the same as a DoLS? Why might you use one form of supervision and not the other? It could be argued that one-to-one care is a form of restriction of liberty as the person is either under continuous observation or care and direction. However, someone with a one-to-one carer may be free to leave (the ward, care home or their own home) at any time and would not be stopped from doing so, merely supported so that their needs are met. Depending on the level of intervention by the carer, this could amount to a restriction meeting the "acid test". The Code of Practice helpfully refers to a sliding scale between <u>restriction</u> and <u>deprivation</u> of liberty, paragraph 6.52:

> *It is difficult to define the difference between actions that amount to a restriction of someone's liberty and those that result in a deprivation of liberty. In recent legal cases, the European Court of Human Rights said that the difference was 'one of degree or intensity, not one of nature or substance'. There must therefore be particular factors in the specific situation of the person concerned which provide the 'degree' or 'intensity' to result in a deprivation of liberty. In practice, this can relate to:*
>
> - *the type of care being provided*
> - *how long the situation lasts*
> - *its effects, or*
> - *the way in a particular situation came about (page 109).*

4 [2020] EWCOP 34, paragraph 50

Key Learning Points

- The potential risks posed to (or by) a person have to be considered carefully and weighed against the underlying principle of adopting the "least restrictive" measures to protect them.
- Each case must be considered individually.
- The distance between <u>restriction</u> and <u>deprivation</u> of liberty is narrow and must be documented in a transparent way that evidences the deliberations of the issues involved.

Case examples to consider

The following are cases to consider in the context of DoLS and are presented to illustrate two common traps that are fallen into by those assessing whether or not the criteria for a DoLS exists, whether a DoLS should be applied for or whether it should be revoked. In such cases, it is common for the assessor to either demonstrate a lack of understanding of the "*hidden nature of ABI-related disabilities*" (Odumuyiwa et al., 2019, p. 170) or be driven by a misguided protection imperative. In the latter circumstance, the driver should always be to implement whatever is the *least restrictive* means of keeping a person safe.

Understanding of the "hidden disability" of acquired brain injury (ABI)

Mr CA was a 65-year-old man with a long history of overuse of alcohol, resulting in Alcohol-Related Brain Damage (ARBD). On previous occasions of having no restrictions, he found himself without money or home because of excessive drinking. He was extremely vulnerable when not protected but appeared, on initial acquaintance, to be completely cognitively intact. He was verbally articulate and appeared to reason his position well. He

vehemently disagreed with being on a DoLS and had been objecting through the Court of Protection, supported by his Solicitor
and IMCA. He was accommodated in a specialist residential unit
which provided him with a structured environment with time-
tabled activities of daily living, including set meal-times, medication slots, domestic tasks and activities as well as opportunities
for social engagement. He had a detailed care plan and was risk
assessed as needing the protection of a DoLS. Support staff, social
worker and family members all felt that he was unable to keep
himself safe but, as he was able to express his views articulately,
this gave a false impression of his ability to reason cogently. He
was verbally plausible at interview, yet none of what he claimed
was matched by action. He would say that he could manage his
medication himself, for example, but numerous carefully structured attempts to skill him up to do so had failed, and he was a
risk of making a serious medication error. He also claimed that
he would be able to find his way around in the local community
and was supported to make plans to do so, on a trial basis. He was
able to find out which bus route and bus number he needed to
take the short trip into town. He was supported to work out how
much money he would need for bus fare. He was encouraged
to ensure that his mobile phone was fully charged before setting
out. The risks of a return to drinking alcohol were fully explained
and understood. He agreed to be followed by support staff, at a
safe distance, as he remained on the DoLS whilst the positive risk
management trial was underway. When put into practice, he was
unable to consistently follow the plan that had been agreed. He,
therefore, met the "*weigh up*", but not the "*use*" element of the
functional test for mental capacity. Without the oversight and
supervision of staff from his placement, **CA** would have returned
to overuse of alcohol in the community, as he made straight for
a pub when he got off the bus. He remained on a DoLS. This is
an exemplar case of an individual being able to "*talk the talk*" but
not able to "*walk the walk*", which is explored in greater detail in
Chapter 5 of this book. There is a reported judgement in a similar
case which makes interesting reading.[5]

5 [2020] EWCOP 34

Mrs CB was a 60-year-old woman with a recent history of drinking heavily within her home. She lived alone but had adult children living in the area, who were unaware of her level of alcohol consumption. She sustained a severe traumatic brain injury when she fell downstairs at home whilst drunk. After several months of orthopaedic treatment, her physical injuries were sufficiently healed for her to regain her lost mobility. Her cognitive deficits were significant, but she retained her verbal communication skills and was verbose, chatty and engaging on a personal level. Visitors to the ward would struggle to identify her as a patient, as she would help out at mealtimes and engage with them in everyday conversation. She would frequently declare that she did not need her bed on the ward, as she was aware that there was a waiting list and that she should just go home as she was *"completely recovered"*. **CB**, however, lacked insight into her difficulties and needs. For example, her family reported that, when they went to check on her house whilst she was in hospital, there were excessive numbers of parcels of clothing being delivered that she was ordering from the ward. They confirmed that she did not need the additional clothes and were concerned that she was buying these without full awareness of her finances or recall of orders she had already made. Of additional concern was the fact that, in preparation for discharge, it came to light that there was a local shop across the road from her home that sold alcohol. She was noted to keep trying to leave the ward to walk home (a distance of several miles involving crossing a motorway). She was placed on a DoLS whilst on the ward, as she was unable to keep herself safe and the concern was that this risk would continue on discharge. She appealed her DoLS and two separate Best Interest Assessors (BIAs) attended her, neither of whom read her clinical notes or spoke to ward staff who knew her well, both of which could be considered to be negligent acts. The BIAs both formed the opinion that she did not need to be on a DoLS, as she was able to articulate the correct answers to questions. However, neither BIA was experienced in acquired brain injury, and both failed to note that **CB** lacked insight into her needs as she was verbally plausible in her responses to questioning. Ward staff appealed the removal of the DoLS, supported by her social worker and family, on both occasions.

A drive to be over-protective

Mr CC was on a DoLS on a neurorehabilitation ward after sustaining a traumatic brain injury in an assault. He had a history of drug misuse and was considered vulnerable. He was noted to be *"pleasant and co-operative"* whilst an inpatient. He had been placed on the DoLS to prevent him from self-discharge from the ward, as there was a real concern that he would return to his previous address, circle of acquaintance and drug use. He underwent detailed neurocognitive testing and clinical interview, and this demonstrated improvement over several months. Individual clinical work with **CC** enabled him to explore his lifestyle pre-injury and he was consistently clear in his expressed view that he had no intention of returning to the same. However, it had been difficult to properly assess whether he was able to turn intention into action. A trial was organised, based on the Multiple Errands Task (Alderman et al., 2003) in the local community, supported by ward staff. **CC** was briefed, prepared and tasked with a series of errands locally, constrained by certain rules, to assess his ability to adapt, think on his feet and alter his actions accordingly. During the task, he was observed to demonstrate a good level of road safety awareness without prompting, to interact appropriately with shop staff and to follow the rules and demands of the tasks with little or no support or prompting from clinical staff who accompanied him. This case demonstrates that, with the appropriate training and support, an individual can have their restrictions to liberty safely removed, despite not being fully recovered and continuing to need 24-hour support going forward.

  Ms CD was a young woman in her twenties who acquired a brain injury in childhood as a result of brain tumours which were surgically resected. She had many physical and cognitive difficulties as a result and was supported in her own home with a 24-hour staffed care package and a clinical therapy team. She was on a DoLS, as her access to food and fluids was restricted due to a swallowing problem (dysphagia) and frequent choking episodes. Following a specialist assessment, she was placed on a level-five diet (minced and moist food only – see International Dysphagia Diet Standardisation Initiative or IDDSI in references) with thickened fluids. She loved her food and care was taken to offer her interesting and palatable food and drink in order to maintain her quality of life. Matters improved over time, and she was able to transition to a level-six diet (soft and bite-sized food only). However, **CD** would frequently attempt to access foods that placed her at risk. For example, on one occasion she purchased a box of breakfast cereal, which consisted of clusters of nuts, oats and freeze-dried fruit, as she wanted to eat this as a snack. She was unable to reason by means of her brain injury and was able to consistently and clearly – occasionally robustly – express her views. What she lacked was the ability to weigh up the information she had about her swallowing difficulties and to use that information in a risk analysis to herself. Staff had to intervene to remove the cereal when it was delivered. A piece of work was undertaken with the Neuropsychologist and the Speech and Language Therapist to educate **CD** about her swallowing difficulties, about her specialist diet and also about the risks involved in not adhering to the agreed-on plan for food and drink. Alongside this work, efforts were made to improve her swallowing mechanism and the situation was kept under review whilst she continued to be constrained by a DoLS. After many months, she was assessed as no longer needing a modified diet, and the DoLS was able to be removed. It had served its purpose as a protective factor for **CD** but only for the minimum amount of time that was needed to enable her to achieve independence in terms of feeding. This case is an example of how DoLS should only ever be used if it is the least restrictive means available to keep a person safe.

4   All Change! Mental Capacity Amendment Act (2019) – Liberty Protection Safeguards

The new Act, which comes into force in April 2022, replaces the current Deprivation of Liberty Safeguards process and is aimed at providing protection for people aged 16 and above who are, or need to be, derived of their liberty. Under these arrangements, a Responsible Body can authorise arrangements amounting to a Deprivation of Liberty. The LPS introduces the following key changes:

- *Three* assessments will form the basis of the new LPS:

  - "Capacity" assessment. The person lacks the relevant capacity to consent to the arrangements.
  - "Medical" assessment (to assess that the person has a mental disorder under the Mental Health Act).
  - "Necessary and proportionate" assessment (to assess whether the arrangements are necessary and proportionate for the prevention of harm to the individual).

- There will be specific duties to consult with the person themselves, carers, IMCA and families.
- Once this process is complete, the evidence will be reviewed before a decision to authorise.
- The approach is more targeted to the individual (with reference to an Approved Mental Capacity Professional).
- There is a new role called Appropriate Person, which will be a non-professional person providing representation and support and who could challenge the LPS.
- The scheme is extended to include 16- and 17-year-olds.
- The LPS covers domestic settings (including shared homes). Strictly speaking, the current DoLS system covers this category but is rarely used and poorly understood.
- Clinical Commissioning Groups, Local Health Boards and National Health Service – NHS- Trusts are now Responsible Bodies (this means that they can authorise the deprivation).

The two systems will run in parallel for the first 12 months of LPS, as there is a gradual transition across for those already in the DoLS system. However, during the period up to the implementation of the LPS, practitioners are exhorted to begin applying the thinking behind the LPS, primarily in terms of consulting widely and also in terms of considering "necessity and proportionality". LPS can be renewed for up to 36 months, so first can be 12 months but thereafter up to 36 months. A person can still challenge their LPS in the Court of Protection under Section 21ZA of the MCA.

What are the main differences between DoLS and LPS?

DoLS	LPS
Special application needed to Court of Protection for 16–17-year-olds.	16–17-year-olds now included in legislation – no special application needed.
Mainly applies to Care Homes (residential and nursing) and Hospitals. Case law* has established that there is a responsibility to ensure that DoLS apply to community too.	Applies to Care Homes, Hospitals, domestic dwellings (included shared homes). Cover extends to those being transported between venues such as Care Home to Day Centre).
Supervisory Body has to provide the person deprived of their liberty with an RPR or IMCA.	No such duty unless the new Responsible Body considers that it is in the person's best interests to do so. Responsible Body is Hospital Manager (if person is an inpatient) or Health Board/Clinical Commissioning Group (if the person has their continuing health care provision funded by these) or the Local Authority.
Urgent and Standard Authorisations	Only Standard Authorisations
Best Interest Assessors automatic right	Approved Mental Capacity Professionals – only if objecting or if in independent hospital
"Best Interests"	"Necessary and Proportional"

* [2016] EWCOP 27

The Code of Practice for the LPS will be combined with that for the Mental Capacity Act which is currently in place. It will have to be published by late autumn 2021 in order to meet with the timetable laid out by the Minister for Care in July 2020. It is expected that the new Code of Practice will contain the following sections, although the headings may change slightly following consultation of the draft document:[6]

- *What is the MCA 2005? (Including an introduction to LPS)*
- *What are the statutory principles and how should they be applied?*
- *How should people be helped to make their own decisions? (Also covering 'How the Person is Involved' and 'Information Rights'.)*
- *How does the Act define a person's capacity to make a decision, and how should capacity be assessed?*
- *What does the Act mean when it talks about "best interests"?*
- *What protection does the Act offer for people providing care or treatment?*
- *What is the role of the Court of Protection? (Also covering 'LPS Court of Protection'.)*
- *What does the Act say about the Lasting Powers of Attorney?*
- *What does the Act say about Deputies?*
- *What is the IMCA Service? (Also covering 'LPS IMCAs'.)*
- *What does the Act say about advance decisions to refuse treatment?*
- *What is a Deprivation of Liberty?*
- *What is the Overall LPS Process? (Also covering 'If I think there is a DoLS')*
- *What is the role of the Responsible Body? (Also covering 'Correct Responsible Body, Responsible Body Oversight of LPS' and 'Cross Border Working'.)*
- *What is the role of the Appropriate Person?*
- *What are the Assessments and Determinations for LPS?*
- *What is the LPS Consultation?*
- *What is the role of the Approved Mental Capacity Professionals (AMCP)?*
- *What is Section 4B, and how is it applied?*
- *How is the LPS system monitored and reported on?*

6 www.mentalcapacitylawandpolicy.org.uk/liberty-protection-safeguards-update-march-2021-what-will-the-code-of-practice-be-likely-to-cover/

- *How does the Act apply to children and young people? (Also covering 'LPS 16–17-Year-Olds'.)*
- *What is the relationship between the Mental Capacity Act and the Mental Health Act of 1983? (Also covering 'Interface between LPS and the MHA'.)*
- *What are the best ways to settle disagreements and disputes about issues covered in the Act? (Also covering 'LPS Challenging Arrangements'.)*
- *What rules govern access to information about a person who lacks the relevant capacity?*
- *How does the Act affect research projects involving a person who lacks the relevant capacity?*

The new process of applying for an LPS is summarised in the following flowchart (although this may change as a result of the consultation process on the new Code of Practice):

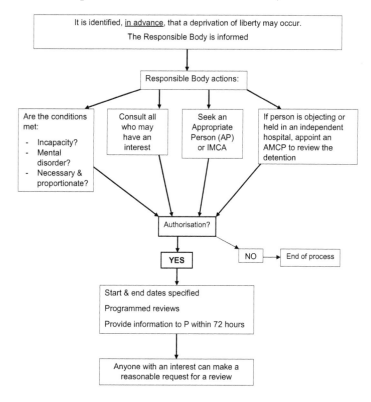

What is good about LPS?

i) Thinking about depriving a person of their liberty will need to be front and centre of any care planning in the future. Plans will need to be made in advance.

ii) Staff will need to be better informed and have a greater awareness of mental capacity.

iii) The scope of depriving a person of the liberty has ostensibly had its reach extended to cover domestic dwellings and also transport between. It is, therefore, transportable with the person. (In reality, this was already possible.)

iv) CCGs and Health Boards will have ownership of the safeguards.

v) Means-tested legal aid will be available to challenges to a LPS and not just limited to those in care homes or hospitals.

What is not so good about LPS?

i) LPS removes a level of protection for the person by taking away the role of RPR. It will be interesting to properly understand the role of the appropriate person who appears to be the substitute and whether they will have the same requirements of them to bring challenges irrespective of their own feelings.

ii) The new guidance (at present) does not give a deadline for completing the assessment for LPS, but it can be assumed that without an LPS it will not be an authorised detention.

iii) There are no specific contact requirements for the Appropriate Person or the IMCA. Under DoLS, they are required to maintain contact. Under LPS, they are only required to "represent and support".

iv) "Best Interests" has vanished as a concept. It has been replaced by "necessary and proportionate". The BIA role has also been removed. (This was a key source of establishing that the DoLS was against the person's wishes.)

v) It may be more difficult for the person's voice of challenge to be heard and acted upon if there are insufficient opportunities to access an IMCA and the appropriate person does not challenge.

What is challenging about new system of LPS?

i) Statutory Children's services will need to get up to speed quickly in terms of understanding and implementing the LPS system.

ii)   Current (planned) arrangements place a heavy reliance on the Code of Practice (rather than legislation) to address any legal concerns that might arise. However, the Code of Practice will have the status of statutory guidance and so should have appropriate weight in the circumstances.

Key Learning Points	• LPS is a replacement for the DoLS in terms of legally depriving a person of their liberty.
	• LPS comes into force in April 2022 and guidance will be provided in a new (combined) Code of Practice for the MCA as a whole.
	• There are significant differences between DoLS and LPS in terms of:
	o Age of person covered;
	o Process of applying for authorisation;
	o Time period of authorisation;
	o Support provided to the person;
	o Places covered;
	o Who to be consulted; and
	o How to object.

References and weblinks for further research/ reading

Alderman, N.; Burgess, P. W.; Knight, C. & Henman, C. (2003) Ecological validity of a simplified version of the multiple errands shopping test. *Journal of the International Neuropsychological Society*, (9), pp. 31–44.

Deprivation of Liberty Safeguards (DoLS). scie.org.uk

For 16 & 17 Year Olds. www.mentalcapacitylawandpolicy.org.uk/deprivation-of-liberty-and-16-17-year-olds-shedinar/

Holloway, M. (2014) How is ABI assessed and responded to in non-specialist settings? Is specialist education required for all social care professionals? *Social Care & Neurodisability*, 5 (4), pp. 201–213.

https://iddsi.org/Framework

In England. www.gov.uk/government/publications/deprivation-of-liberty-safeguards-forms-and-guidance

In Wales. https://gov.wales/mental-capacity-act-deprivation-liberty-guidance-and-forms

Liberty Protection Safeguards: New Factsheets: Mental Capacity Law and Policy.

Mental Capacity Law and Policy.

Moore, S.; Wotus, R.; Norman, A.; Holloway, M. & Dean, J. (2019) Behind the cloak of competence: Brain injury and mental capacity legislation. *The Journal of Adult Protection*, *21* (4), pp. 201–218.

Norman, A.; Holloway, M.; Odumuyiwa, T.; Kennedy, M.; Forrest, H. & Suffield, F. (2020) Accepting what we do not know: A need to improve professional understanding of brain injury in the UK. *Health & Social Care in the Community*, *28*, pp. 2037–2049.

Odumuyiwa, T.; Kennedy, M.; Norman, A.; Holloway, M.; Suffield, F.; Forrest, H. & Dicks, H. (2019) Improving access to social care services following acquired brain injury: A needs analysis. *Journal of Long-Term Care*, pp. 164–175.

www.gov.uk/government/publications/deprivation-of-liberty-safeguards-supreme-court-judgments

Chapter 4

What is the "general defence"?

1 Section 5 of the Mental Capacity Act (2005)

Section 5 of the MCA provides protection from liability for those who provide care/assistance for those who lack capacity for issues such as:

- Assistance with dressing,
- Having a shower/wash, and
- Entering a person's home to provide care/cleaning.

It is known as the "general defence".
The Act allows necessary acts in connection with care or treatment to take place as if a person who lacks capacity to consent had consented to them and absolves them of the civil or criminal liability that might otherwise be present. For example, providing intimate personal care could be deemed an assault (criminal act), or entering someone's house to deliver their shopping could be considered a form of trespass (criminal act). People providing care of this sort do not therefore need to get formal authority to act. It is important to understand that, although Section 5 offers protection from liability so that staff can act in connection with the person's care or treatment, it does **not** allow for staff to make decisions regarding care or treatment on behalf of the person who lacks capacity. (Other sections of the MCA provide for this, such as those that provide for Welfare Deputies.)

DOI: 10.4324/9781003205210-4

Section 5 of the MCA states that

1) *If a person ("D") does an act in connection with the care or treatment of another person ("P"), the act is one to which this section applies if –*

   a) *before doing the act, D takes reasonable steps to establish whether P lacks capacity in relation to the matter in question, and*

   b) *when doing the act, D reasonably believes –*

      (i) *that P lacks capacity in relation to the matter, and*

      (ii) *that it will be in P's best interests for the act to be done.*

2) *D does not incur any liability in relation to the act that he would not have incurred if P –*

   a) *had had capacity to consent in relation to the matter, and*

   b) *had consented to D's doing the act.*

Section 5, however, does not protect the person undertaking the act from civil liability for loss, damage or negligence.

Who is protected by Section 5?

- Members of the person's family providing care;
- Paid care workers;
- Health staff (nurses, health and social care workers; physiotherapists, radiographers, for example) and social care staff, and
- Others who may occasionally be involved in the care or treatment of a person who lacks capacity to consent (for example, ambulance staff, housing workers, police officers and volunteer support workers).

It is important to consider whether the person carrying out the act is the right person and is doing so at the right time for the person being cared for. For example, if the intervention involves personal care, is it possible for a member of staff of the same gender to carry out the care? If there is a member of staff who speaks the same language, might they be better placed to provide the care or intervention? If the person is unwell, can the intervention wait until they are feeling better? If the staff is about to wash the person's hair, is this done more safely in a shower or a bath, and which might the person prefer if asked?

Key Learning Points	• If you are required to carry out day-to-day acts of health or social care for a person in connection with your duties, and you reasonably believe that the person lacks capacity to consent, you are protected from civil suit or criminal prosecution by Section 5 of the MCA.
	• Make sure that the care or intervention is carried out by the right person, at the best time and in the most appropriate place.

2   *What* is covered by the "general defence"?

The acts that are carried out must be considered to be in the person's best interests and something to which they would consent if they retained the mental capacity to do so. Examples of these acts are provided in Chapter 6 of the Code of Practice.

Personal care:

- Helping with washing, dressing or personal hygiene;
- Helping with eating and drinking;
- Helping with communication;
- Helping with mobility (moving around);
- Helping someone take part in education, social or leisure activities;
- Going into a person's home to drop off shopping or to see if they are alright;
- Doing the shopping or buying necessary goods with the person's money;
- Arranging household services (for example, arranging repairs or maintenance for gas and electricity supplies);
- Providing services that help around the home (such as homecare or meals on wheels);

- Undertaking actions related to community care services (for example, day care, residential accommodation or nursing care); and
- Helping someone to move home (including moving property and clearing the former home).

Healthcare and treatment:

- Carrying out diagnostic examinations and tests (to identify an illness, condition or other problem);
- Providing professional medical, dental and similar treatment;
- Giving medication;
- Taking someone to hospital for assessment or treatment;
- Providing nursing care (whether in hospital or in the community);
- Carrying out any other necessary medical procedures (for example, taking a blood sample) or therapies (for example, physiotherapy or chiropody); and
- Providing care in an emergency.

Whilst that might seem straightforward, the Code of Practice points out that there may be a situation where the person for whom the care is being provided might not have consented or might not have chosen that particular intervention for themselves. This is considered further in terms of the doctrine of necessity.

On occasion, it may become necessary to use physical restraint on a person who lacks capacity to carry out an act of care or treatment. In such situations, all other reasonable actions to defuse or de-escalate must have been considered and/or implemented. Restraint should only be used if there is no other realistic option to prevent harm to the person. The amount or type of restraint used needs to be least restrictive, proportionate (to the likelihood and seriousness of potential harm) and used for the minimum amount of time that it takes to keep the person safe from harm. As restraint could be classed as a deprivation of liberty, careful and serious consideration needs to be given to this line of action.

Key   •   Many day-to-day acts of care are covered within
Learning   the terms of the general defence that can be
Points   considered collectively under the headings of
                      personal care, healthcare and treatment.

              •   Separate consideration needs to be given to
                   those acts of care or treatment that the person
                   is unlikely to have consented to if they had the
                   mental capacity to do so.

              •   Careful consideration needs to be given
                   to the use of restraint, as this needs to be
                   proportionate to the risk, for the purpose
                   of preventing harm and only applied for the
                   minimum amount of time. There are implications
                   for depriving the person of their liberty.

3   Doctrine of Necessity (Law Lords *Re F*)[1]

An intervention, without the consent of the person, can be
considered to be lawful if it is deemed <u>necessary</u>. The common
law "doctrine of necessity" pre-dates the Mental Capacity Act,
as it was established in the seminal case of *Re F* in 1989, but
the principles which underpin the doctrine apply within the
framework of the MCA, nonetheless.

It is important to understand that, "*emergency is not the same
as necessity*" (*Re F*, paragraph 565). Lord Brandon stated that
a best interests' intervention is lawful under the doctrine of
necessity "*if, it is carried out in order either to save their lives, or to
ensure improvement or prevent deterioration in their physical or mental
health*" (Re F, paragraph 551). This suggests that it only applies
to medical emergencies. As such, in an <u>emergency</u> situation,
a patient may be treated without consent under the doctrine
of necessity, as long as there is a necessity to act, and it is not

1 [1989] 2 All ER 545

practicable or possible to communicate with the patient. The action taken should be no more than is immediately necessary and in the best interests of the patient. This can only take place if there is no Advanced Decision to Refuse Treatment (ADRT) in place, or if the treating staff consider the ADRT not to be valid or relevant to the treatment in question. This approach appears to suggest that the scope of the doctrine of necessity is narrow.

However, *"the court* (in *Re F*) *also held that the doctrine includes decisions made in everyday life, as well as serious situations . . . .demonstrat(ing) how broad the common law doctrine of necessity can be drawn"*. Gooding & Flynn (2015, p. 259). The authors were referring to paragraph 566 of *Re F* where Lord Goff stated, *"when the state of affairs is permanent, or semi-permanent, action properly taken to preserve the life, health or well-being of the assisted person may well transcend such measures as surgical operation or substantial medical treatment and may extend to include such humdrum matters as routine medical or dental treatment, even simple care such as dressing and undressing and putting to bed . . . . . . it is the necessity itself which provides the justification for the intervention"* (paragraph 567).

Therefore, it could be argued that the "general defence" (Section 5) of the MCA represents an attempt to narrow the scope of the doctrine of necessity, to protect the human rights of the individual. *"However, this legislative provision is still drawn very broadly and allows for decisions to be made in situations which are not emergency situations . . ."* Gooding & Flynn (2015, p. 259).

As with many aspects of the MCA, there is a constant balance to be struck between autonomy and protection for the individual subject to its clauses. In the situation of assessing to treat, the clinician needs to follow a transparent process once a lack of capacity is established. In that context, it is worthwhile considering the view of the Law Lord Jauncey in *Re F* which is reported as follows:

> *There are four stages in the treatment of a patient, whether competent or incompetent. The <u>first</u> is to diagnose the relevant condition. The <u>second</u> is to determine whether the condition merits treatment. The <u>third</u> is to determine what the merited treatment should be.*

The fourth is to carry out the chosen form of merited treatment. In the case of a longterm incompetent, convenience to those charged with his care should never be a justification for the decision to treat. However, if such persons take the decision in relation to the second and third stages (supra) solely in his best interests and if their approach to and execution of all four stages is such as would be adopted by a responsible body of medical opinion skilled in the particular field of diagnosis and treatment concerned, they will have done all that is required of them and their actings will not be subject to challenge as being unlawful. (paragraph 572)

What kind of clinical presentations might be subject to the consideration of the doctrine of necessity?

- Patients who refuse treatment that is considered to be necessary and proportionate
- Patients who abscond (or attempt to self-discharge against medical advice when assessments or treatments are incomplete, and their health and physical integrity may remain at risk)
- Patients suffering from long term conditions that impair their ability to make decisions. This might include the dementias and similar neurodegenerative conditions, all of which exert a cognitive effect and have the potential to impair decision-making.
- Patients suffering from temporary lack of capacity due to intoxication, delirium, or reduced level of consciousness.
- Patients at the end of life who wish to refuse further treatment even when this is considered to be medically necessary.
- Patients whose mental health condition impairs their ability to make decisions such as when in an acute phase of a chronic condition such as schizophrenia or bipolar disorder.

The following flowchart summarises the overlap between the application of the doctrine of necessity with the General Defence of section 5 of the MCA.

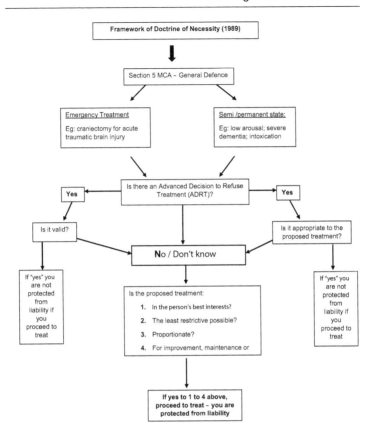

Framework of Doctrine of Necessity (1989)

Section 5 MCA – General Defence

Emergency Treatment

Eg: craniectomy for acute traumatic brain injury

Semi /permanent state:

Eg: low arousal; severe dementia; intoxication

Is there an Advanced Decision to Refuse Treatment (ADRT)?

Yes

Yes

Is it valid?

Is it appropriate to the proposed treatment?

No / Don't know

If "yes" you are not protected from liability if you proceed to treat

If "yes" you are not protected from liability if you proceed to treat

Is the proposed treatment:

1. In the person's best interests?

2. The least restrictive possible?

3. Proportionate?

4. For improvement, maintenance or

If yes to 1 to 4 above, proceed to treat – you are protected from liability

Key Learning Points	•	The common law "doctrine of necessity" underpins the general defence in section 5 of MCA.
	•	It applies to both emergency situations and those where the person's condition which prevents them from consenting is semi or fully permanent.
	•	If there is a valid and appropriate ADRT in place, and the treating clinician knows about it, they are not protected from liability if they proceed to treat anyway.

- If there is not a valid or appropriate ADRT, the treating clinician must proceed in line with considerations as to best interests, least restrictive, proportionate and that there is a clinical justification for treating.

4 Wilful Mistreatment and Neglect

Section 44 of the Mental Capacity Act (2005) has introduced the offences of ill treatment or neglect against the person who has the care of the person who lacks capacity or is appointed to act on their behalf, such as an Attorney or Deputy. If the person is convicted, they are liable to imprisonment for up to five years or a maximum fine, or both. The acts to the person are defined as deliberate (wilful). Some published examples are:

- A Manager was convicted of four counts of ill-treating a person without capacity against three victims at a residential care home.[2]
- A senior carer in a registered care home was convicted of two offences under Section 44 and sentenced to consecutive three- and six-month sentences of imprisonment.[3]
- Four members of staff at a care home were charged with wilfully neglecting one of their residents.[4]

5 Case Examples to consider

DA (This case is cited as an example of a permanent state of necessity to treat under general defence)

Mr DA was a 30-year-old man who had sustained a very severe traumatic brain injury as a result of a motorcycle accident. He was several years post-injury and required full, 24-hour care, including full mechanical and staff support for all transfers

---

2 *R v Dunn* [2010] EWCA Crim 2935
3 *R v Heaney* [2011] EWCA Crim 2682
4 *R v Turbill* [2013] EWCA Crim 1422, [2013] MHLO 70

and mobility. He had significant ongoing health issues including post-traumatic epilepsy which required medication for frequent seizures. He was unable to communicate verbally and was fully supported by staff, who became familiar with his gestures, body language and facial expressions. He was provided with an AAC (Augmentative and Alternative Communication device, which replaces speech or writing for those unable to communicate by other means) but struggled to use it at a fast enough place to communicate fluently. He frequently chose not to use the AAC, despite prompting and support.

DA lacked insight and awareness into his brain injury and would insist that he could walk unaided and would ride a motorcycle again, live independently and care for his children without any support or formal help. Despite consistent interventions by both his family and by clinical and support staff to assist with awareness of his needs over many months, no progress was made. None of his aspirations was realistic because of the extent and severity of his brain and physical injuries.

DA had a PEG (Percutaneous Endoscopic Gastrostomy). This is a means of introducing food, fluids and medicines directly into the stomach by passing a thin tube through the skin and into the stomach) in situ, as he had an unreliable swallow and it had been demonstrated on videofluorosopy assessment that he silently aspirated with all oral intake. As a result, **DA** received all of his fluids, food and medication through his PEG. He often expressed unhappiness with this, as he missed the taste and texture of food. For periods of time, he would refuse all intake, even through his PEG, as a means of communicating his wishes. Neuropsychological assessment of his behaviours concluded that as the only form of control that **DA** could exert was to refuse food, drink and medicines, he would use this as a means of communicating his key wishes, which were to walk again and to eat a normal diet, also referred to as a level-seven (regular) diet (according to the International Dysphagia Diet Standardisation Initiative – see references).

Work was undertaken with **DA** to assist with introducing some oral taste and texture (not for nutritional purposes) to improve his quality of life. There was a specific behavioural management guideline drawn up to ensure that all risks were minimised, such as only providing the taste experience when he was rested, settled and in a quiet environment. Despite the fact that he greatly enjoyed the experience, it was not possible to safely increase the intake to ensure that he was receiving adequate nutrition and hydration and also adhering to his prescribed medications. His PEG was essential for these purposes. He continued to object to having a PEG.

A Mental Capacity Assessment was undertaken with **DA** in which his views were ascertained in terms of his wishes, his beliefs and his understanding of the need for his PEG. This involved ensuring that **DA** understood:

- The fact that he had sustained a very severe traumatic brain injury;
- The fact that he was unable to swallow food, drink and medicines safely (as a result of his brain injury) without risking taking these down into his lungs and, as a result, risking a chest infection, or worse;
- The fact that he had post-traumatic epilepsy;
- The fact that he needed to have regular medication to control his seizures;
- The fact that without his anti-epileptic medication he ran the risk of experiencing seizures and that these could be life-threatening; and
- That his medication could only safely be delivered via PEG.

The assessment demonstrated that **DA** could not understand that he needed his medication. He did not accept that he had seizures or that without the regular administration of his medication his health would be at significant risk. He continued to refuse his medication by his PEG and would physically resist its administration.

A Best Interests process considered that he absolutely had to have his anti-epileptic medication because of the risk to life. A range of options had to be considered. One option was to continue to try to verbally persuade **DA** to take his medication. This had only been intermittently successful to date and had led to him objecting to certain members of staff entering his room as he came to associate them with battles over medication. A second option was to consider administering his medication covertly, without his consent or knowledge, following strict protocols to do so. The second option was favoured as the least restrictive and the least distressing for **DA**. There is clear national guidance for the covert administration of medicines (Both NICE and CQC provide guidance) and this was closely followed, including obtaining advice from a pharmacist. The plan was recorded and implemented with regular reviews in place.

Key Learning Points	In some cases, there may be a permanent "necessity" to treat under the terms of general defence in Section 5 of the MCA. In all cases where treatment has to proceed, it needs to be the least restrictive and also in the best interests of the person, according to all key stakeholders.

DB (this case is cited as an example of where the doctrine of necessity was considered for a person refusing treatment but where they were assisted and supported to regain the capacity to drive their own treatment plan)

Ms DB was a 20-year-old young woman who had sustained a traumatic brain injury in a road traffic collision. Neuroradiological reporting had indicated extensive injuries within the brain which would classify her injury as "very severe".

She had a period of inpatient acute neurorehabilitation followed by a placement at a slower-stream rehabilitation unit for adults with acquired brain injury. However, she had absconded from the latter and made the long train journey home to her family, despite being considered unsafe to travel independently.

DB was described by her treating Multi-Disciplinary Team (MDT) as presenting with the classical "frontal lobe paradox" in which the individual appears competent and capable but is unable to apply their knowledge in the situations where it is required. She was described as having "rigid" and "concrete" thinking, demonstrating an inability to reason, to consider or to weigh up information from different perspectives. It was also said that she lacked insight into either her injuries or her needs which followed from it. She refused medication prescribed by her treating Neuropsychiatrist, which included a mood-stabilising drug in order to balance and regulate her explosive mood changes.

An experienced Brain Injury Case Manager was appointed who, in turn, instructed a private team of neurorehabilitation specialists, including Clinical Neuropsychology, Neuro-Occupational Therapy and Neuro-Physiotherapy. The clinical team met with **DB**, both individually and as a team, to formulate rehabilitation goals with her. For example, she had not been able to undertake many activities of daily living without prompting and support at her placement, and she was keen to live as "normal" a life as possible. **DB** had only limited insight into the impact of her traumatic brain injury, and, therefore, her ongoing need for support and rehabilitation. The starting point was a complex assessment, involving her, her family, and her treating team, of **DB**'s capacity to make decisions about residence, care and treatment. The key theme of the process was to provide **DB** with information which could be used to guide her insight into her needs in order to augment her ability to make informed decisions.

DB had significant and substantial cognitive impairments as a result of her very severe traumatic brain injury, including extensive damage to the frontal areas of her brain involved in awareness, taking new information into memory and evaluating information in the process of decision-making.

The immediate outcome of the assessment was that **DB** lacked the mental capacity to make informed decisions about her care and treatment but was able (with considerable assistance) to decide upon her residence. In this case, it was possible to separate these, but often the two are conflated. The next steps involved a period of intensive support to provide **DB** with information, in a format that she could understand and remember with prompting, in relation to her daily support needs. Her family were instrumental in supporting this period of intervention. **DB** was provided with a structured routine, with a clear balance between activities she needed to do (such as laundry) with activities she enjoyed doing (such as exercise). The routine enabled her to schedule periods of regular rest which helped with her sleep and mood difficulties, and she became much more settled. It came to light that her refusal of neurorehabilitation stemmed from her feelings of being overwhelmed by so many professionals all wanting to work with her at the same time and expecting her to make progress on all fronts. She had previously voted with her feet and had established a pattern of regular non-engagement in sessions she did not see the point in. The MDT worked closely with **DB** to ensure that the approach was revised to focus on what was essential and accepted by **DB** rather that what the MDT considered to be ideal for her, which she had consistently rejected. Following a period of consultation and involvement of both **DB** and her family, whose views she valued and respected, **DB** was considered to have regained the mental capacity to decide on her care and treatment and became an active, if somewhat occasionally reluctant, participant in a programme of neurorehabilitation. Like many adults with brain injury who participate in community-based rehabilitation, **DB** found that support within the home was intrusive and disrupted her enjoyment of family life. The key is to strike a balance, an approach which was successful in the case of **DB** as it enabled rehabilitation to continue, which was to her benefit given her continued potential for improvement.

Key Learning Points	In some cases where at face value it may appear that the doctrine of necessity leads to the urgent need to treat, with careful consideration and with the treating team in agreement, there may be sufficient time to engage the person in the process to the point where they regain the mental capacity to decide on their treatment.

Reflections of a professional: specialist brain injury nursing home deputy manager (Rachael Thomas)

All residents admitted here without capacity are subject to a Best Interests (BI) decision prior to admission. When the patient is admitted to us, we are made to repeat this prior to submitting a DoLS. This I think is inefficient and unnecessary, as it could have been done the day before. It feels as though each organisation does not trust the other in terms of capacity and best interests.

*For a number of years, staff were expected to conduct BI for washing, dressing and similar tasks, but this has thankfully stopped in recent years. Most of our residents are admitted with a DNACPR (Do Not Attempt Cardio Pulmonary Resuscitation), usually not long prior to admission to us, and is usually as part of the "not for re-admission" or "escalation of treatment" decisions. We are told to **redo** the MCA/BI. In terms of DNACPR, this should be **reviewed** on a change of setting, yes, but revisiting the BI process again seem a waste of resources and, again, unnecessary.*

Many other organisations just do not seem to understand what decisions require a BI and what do not. For example, recently a DoLS assessment was granted with the condition that an MCA/BI was completed for a lady with a PEG, as her medication is delivered through on the basis that represented a covert administration. I completely disagreed so did not complete this and was vindicated when the DoLS went back in for renewal; the next DoLS Assessor removed it, as they agreed this was not necessary.

We have recently been asked to complete MCA/BI for COVID testing. We are not asked to do this for any other medical tests we do such as bloods or swabs. I do not understand why these are not classed, and treated, as the same.

We have also been asked to complete MCA/BI for patients that have PEG tubes in. We have challenged this as "what is the decision to be made here?" People who require PEG tubes who lack capacity again have this decision made in their best interests prior to insertion. Why would this be revisited just to use them? The only time we would reassess capacity and complete BI is if we were looking to withdraw feeding.

Assessments and BI we routinely complete are for use of bed rails, lap belts, sensor mats and anything that restricts liberty, covert medication, access to food (if over-/underweight), any new treatment required if in our care home at the time, finance for Power Of Attorney, 1:1 care and support. I think organisations are over-cautious in fear of litigation.

I generally think that people just do not understand what is covered within the MCA and what is the threshold for an MCA/BI. I think more definition is required for Health Care Professionals on General Defence. In my experience, most qualified nurses are poorly trained and ill-equipped to conduct these assessments. I commonly hear nurses stating, "X doesn't have capacity", which I respond to with "capacity in terms of what?". Many still don't understand that capacity is decision-specific.

Head of nursing (Sharron Price)

From the NHS perspective, we can have a variety of individuals who may at some time in their journey require the support of the Mental Capacity Act. Understanding varies greatly and in general will be carrying out acts on patients who may not be able to consent using the "general defence" but without the true knowledge of what they are able to do under this cover. An example may be taking blood pressure or observations; if a patient held out their arm, then the team would consider this as implied consent but without consideration to if the patient is able to truly consent to the investigation or observation.

Often on busy acute wards, you will see the patient's wishes and needs over-ridden by the routine and tasks required rather than a person-focused approach, taking time to offer choices and encourage participation in decision-making around care. This can lead to the care staff undertaking interventions such as washing, feeding, giving medication, etc., where the patient is actively objecting and little consideration may be given to the level of restraint required to undertake the intervention or if there is a less restrictive option.

One example of this is where a frail older male patient with mild dementia was described as being aggressive and resistive to care; nursing staff were unable to wash and dress him in the morning without him shouting, hitting out and getting very angry. When sitting down with the patient to explore how our approaches to care could better support him, it became evident that he was not a "morning person" and would never get out of bed before he had a cup of tea and breakfast. By understanding his usual routine, the care approach was able to be adapted to allow him time to wake up, have a cup of tea and get out of bed in his own time. The incidents of aggression significantly reduced and levels of restrictions with them. During this care episode whilst the patient was deprived of his liberty under the DoLS safeguards, there was no level of restraint agreed within the best interest assessment; the nurses were undertaking the care interventions under what could be viewed as "general defence"; however, the level of restraint applied could arguable not be the least restrictive approach.

There are policies in place in most NHS environments which will support staff for interventions such as giving medication where the person may be resistive but lack capacity to understand the risks involved, and you will often see Covert Medication policies employed in these cases.

In summary, the knowledge and skills of the application of the Mental Capacity Act varies greatly across all areas of in-patient care, with some wards still operating on the premise that if the patient is not actively trying to leave, then there is no deprivation, whilst other areas will have a good understanding and knowledge of the Mental Capacity Act and the safeguards required.

References/links for further reading

Gooding, P. & Flynn, E. (2015) Querying the call to introduce mental capacity testing to mental health law: Does the doctrine of necessity provide an alternative? *Laws, 4* (2), pp. 245–271.

https://assets.publishing.service.gov.uk/government/uploads/system/uploads/attachment_data/file/921428/Mental-capacity-act-code-of-practice.pdf

https://iddsi.org/Framework

The Mental Capacity Act in Emergency Medicine Practice. (2017) www.rcem.ac.uk/docs/RCEM%20Guidance/RCEM%20Mental%20Capacity%20Act%20in%20EM%20Practice%20-%20Feb%202017.pdf

www.cqc.org.uk/guidance-providers/adult-social-care/covert-administration-medicines

www.nice.org.uk/about/nice-communities/social-care/quick-guides/giving-medicines-covertly

www.researchgate.net/publication/279248380_Querying_the_Call_to_Introduce_Mental_Capacity_Testing_to_Mental_Health_Law_Does_the_Doctrine_of_Necessity_Provide_an_Alternative

Complex and challenging issues in MCA from the frontal lobe paradox, giving evidence in the Court of Protection to how to deal with an impasse in best interests

> The person with frontal lobe damage rarely has any insight into it –
> how can the "I" know that it is changed? It has nothing to compare
> itself with. How can I know if I am the same person today as I was
> yesterday? I can only assume that I am. Our selves are unique and
> can only know ourselves as we are now, in the immediate present.
>
> (Marsh, 2017, p. 12)

1   What do we mean by "frontal lobe involvement"?

It can be seen from Chapter 2, where the issue of decision-making
is explored, that the frontal lobes play a key role as they help
to balance one's impulses with the ability to reason. When this
system is working well, it could be argued that we make reasonable, rational, explainable decisions – most of the time, at least.
However, this chapter is concerned with how decision-making
can be compromised when the frontal brain systems are impaired
or injured. This is referred to as executive dysfunction.

In practice, this is often described as the person who is being
assessed as being able to respond to the assessor with the correct, concrete, knowledge but then be manifestly unable to
apply that knowledge in the moment of decision-making. This
is attributed to the "hidden nature" of ABI-related disabilities
(Odumuyiwa et al., 2019) such that professionals without specialist knowledge or training in brain injury conduct *"flawed*

DOI: 10.4324/9781003205210-5

assessment processes which are based upon the verbal output of the assessed person, not their actual functioning in practice" (UKABIF, 2019).

The trade-off that can be difficult to understand is that between "*online*" and "*offline*" awareness, also described as the disconnect between "*knowing*" and "*doing*" that was first described in the 1960s (Teuber, 1964). More recently, George & Gilbert (2018) referred to such individuals as being "*good in theory but poor in practice*" (p. 59).

The NICE Guidance on Decision-Making and Mental Capacity offers the following advice:

> *Practitioners should be aware that it may be more difficult to assess capacity in people with executive dysfunction, for example, people with traumatic brain injury. Structured assessments of capacity for individuals in this group (for example, by way of interview) may therefore need to be supplemented by real-world observation of the person's functioning and decision-making ability in order to provide the assessor with a complete picture of an individual's decision-making ability* (2018, paragraph 1.4.19).

This echoes the advice of experienced Neuropsychologists, who suggest that:

> *It is unwise, even negligent, to form opinions on how test performance is likely to influence everyday behaviour, without carefully interviewing those with direct experience of the person's real-world behaviour over a period of time* (Wood & Bigler, 2017, p. 93).

The importance of this approach is to avoid being erroneously convinced by the "*cloak of competence*" giving the false appearance of capacity (Moore et al., 2019, p. 207). The Code of Practice describes this as occurring when "*the impairment or disturbance leads to a person making a specific decision without . . . using the information they have been given*" and that they "*might make impulsive decisions regardless of information they have been given or their understanding of it*" (paragraphs 4.12 & 4.22). The Code goes further with the caution that "*skills and behaviour do not necessarily reflect the person's capacity to make specific decisions. The fact that someone had good social or language skills, polite behaviour or*

good manners doesn't necessarily mean they understand the informa-
tion or are able to weigh it up" (paragraph 4.49).

Moore et al. (2019) suggest that *"the assessor must therefore*
develop strategies for probing beyond the façade" (p. 3) and *"should*
probe for the ability to have effective online awareness of deficits and
awareness" (p. 30). This is taken further by Cameron & Codling
(in press), who support the "articulate/demonstrate" approach
to assessing individuals with such difficulties. This requires the
person to both tell you what they would do and also to demonstrate the same in practice, thus encouraging a performative
aspect to the capacity assessment.

Key   There is a significant minority of individuals who, as a
Learning   result of damage to their front-of-brain systems (also
Points   sometimes referred to as executive dysfunction or
                frontal lobe paradox) are unable to put into practice
                what they have understood or remembered in order
                to use that information to make a capacitous decision.
                Assessors should not rely solely on interview with the
                person and should seek other sources of information,
                including a practical component to the assessment and
                the views of reliable collateral informants.

2   What does it mean to *"use or weigh "* when making a decision?

Moore et al. (2019) reviewed a range of contested mental capacity cases in the courts and identified that, *"it was the weighing up*
and using that appeared to be the one that was most noted to be cited as
the reason for perceived lack of capacity" (p. 202). The authors go on
to report an experienced case manager, who said that:

> *I have found that my clients can sometimes understand information given*
> *to them about a significant decision and can take part in a discussion of*
> *pros and cons about the decision but are not able to take those discussions*
> *into account when they are alone and in the heat of the moment* (p. 207).

Ruck Keene et al. (2019) examined a significant number of cases that had come before the Court of Protection and reported that in 21 of 23 cases where a functional inability was reported as the reason for lacking capacity, the inability to "*use or weigh*" was cited as one of the reasons, and in seven cases, it was the <u>only</u> reason given. It is noted that "*it is not uncommon to be able to factually understand information while being unable to use or weigh it*" (p. 67).

The Court of Protection has had several key cases before it in which the factor of executive dysfunction has been considered to render the person unable to "*use or weigh*" the key information pertinent to the decision. In a case where the Court was being asked to consider whether a person had the mental capacity to decide whether to live with her husband or not, Parker J held that "*now she is unable to use and weigh the information because of the compromise in her executive functioning*".[1]

A further case relied on the evidence of a Neuropsychologist (Professor Narinder Kapur) in advising that:

> *People with executive functioning deficits . . . may be okay but they may have difficulty in selecting the right bits of information and using them in the right context. . . . [P] has not been able to bring to mind information that it is important to know in the moment to make the relevant decision.*[2]

In a much more recent case, The Honourable Mr Justice Cobb, who was hearing a case of an elderly gentleman who was medically fit for discharge but extremely resistant to leave hospital, concluded that:

> *He is unable to retain abstract information about his future potential residence arrangements and care needs even when encouraged to do so, and is further unable to use and weigh the information relevant to the decision about his future residence and care.*[3]

---

1 [2014] EWCOP 14, paragraph 92
2 [2019] EWCOP 14, paragraph 36
3 [2021] EWCOP 30, paragraph 45

This begs the question as to how much information one should share with the person needing to make the decision, if their clinical presentation is such that they are manifestly unable to use or weigh up the information that they are given. At first glance, the guiding principle should be that any information that relates to them should be shared with them in whatever format best meets their needs. However, each case should be reviewed in terms of its own particular, individual circumstance. Consider the following case example:

Mr EA sustained a severe brain injury in a motorcycle accident. One of the effects of the accident was Organic Personality Disorder (OPD), in which he became suspicious to the point of paranoia and would obsess about how he believed that those supporting him were lying to him and stealing his money. His thinking was rigid and inflexible, and he only understood matters in concrete terms. He had marked cognitive deficits which meant that even when he was provided with the information he requested, he would quickly forget both the content of the information and the fact that it had been shared with him. He would become easily agitated and transition quickly to verbal aggression which involved making threats to others. One of the issues he would obsess about would be money. He had been provided with a Court-Appointed Deputy on the grounds that he lacked the mental capacity to manage his property and affairs. However, arrangements had been put in place to encourage him to manage a small amount of money for day-to-day expenditure as well as involving him in larger household transactions. He would contact the Deputy several times a day demanding both information and money for purchases he had already made and forgotten about. He would become agitated and abusive and state that he wished for his Deputy and Case Manager to both be removed on the grounds that they were spending his money wastefully. Attempts were made to reach out to his wife both to support her, as she was also on the receiving end of the verbal aggression, but also to seek her assistance in communicating in the best way for **EA**. However, it emerged that she was afraid of him, and she declined further contact in fear of retribution from him. In this case, there were many complex issues to address, but from an information-sharing point-of-view, it became clear that whatever the Deputy and Case Manager did in terms of supporting **EA** with his finances, it served to feed his agitation and suspicion. If they withheld information on the grounds that it would upset him for no useful purpose, that led to difficulties. If they gave information and attempted to explain and support, that also led to difficulties. **EA** had been prescribed medication by his Consultant Neuropsychiatrist but stopped taking it which served to increase his paranoid ideation. His lack of ability to use the information he was regularly given in order to weigh up the issues that were in front of him made it challenging to support him meaningfully in terms of decision-making. If information was withheld, **EA** would refuse to engage. If information was given, **EA** would misinterpret or forget it and become difficult to support because of his challenging behaviour.

The case of **EA** is unusual but not atypical of those who sustain either injury or damage to the systems that are mediated by the front of their brain. However, in cases where it is possible to engage with the person, a useful means of assessing real-life skills where frontal lobe systems have been damaged is within the Multiple Errands Task (Shallice & Burgess, 1991) which has also been adapted for use in a hospital setting (Knight et al., 2002). The purpose was to devise a test of planning and multi-tasking that was ecologically valid (i.e., not carried out in a formal testing situation but in a real-life situation). The original test involved the person being set up with a series of tasks to be carried out in a local shopping centre, within certain rules and time constraints. The latter was a modified version for use within a hospital setting for patients who were too unwell or unsafe to be assessed in the local community. Knight et al. (2002) argue that:

> *Links between assessment and rehabilitation may be more obvious when the former is undertaken within "real life" contexts* (p. 233).

An example of the test in a community setting might be as follows:

Buy the following items in town

- Small brown loaf
- Packet of plasters
- Birthday card
- Bar of chocolate
- Single light bulb
- Key ring

Find out the following information

- What is the headline from today's *Daily Mail*?
- What is the closing time of Boots?
- What is the price of a pint of milk in Tesco?
- How many shops did you see today that sell televisions?

Rules

- Spend as little money as possible
- Take as little time as possible
- Shops can only be entered once
- Shops can only be entered to buy something
- Do the tasks in any order
- Meet me at Costa Coffee 20 minutes after you have started and tell me the time

Hospital-based tasks might be more straightforward but still conform to the structure of needing to plan the tasks while sticking to both rule and time constraints, such as:

- Nurse-led trips to hospital shop for a single purpose;
- Drawing up a plan for the patient to manage their own medication with reducing prompts; and
- Planning for the patient to increase their self-care (Personal Hygiene Routine) with reducing prompts.

Key Learning Points

- Frontal lobe systems are critical to informed decision-making (particularly "using and weighing up").
- Patients with frontal lobe paradox (or executive dysfunction) can sometimes talk the talk but cannot walk the walk.
- Don't _assume_ that the patient has preserved or full insight, no matter what they say. Patients with frontal lobe paradox can be verbally plausible, but this may be just a "_cloak of competence_".
- Don't rely solely on interview with the patient. Make sure that you also:

  o Speak to staff who know the person well,
  o Speak to family who are close to the person,
  o Read the clinical notes made by professionals who have worked with the person, and
  o Observe the person engaged in day-to-day tasks.

There is evidence from the Court of Protection that this approach is both acknowledged and valued. In a very recent case,[4] the judge had to decide whether the person had the capacity to conduct the proceedings and to manage his property and affairs. The Neuropsychologist who gave expert evidence to the court had included the Multiple Errands Task as part of her assessment. The observational evidence was considered vital in terms of the final determination by bringing together interview and observation data to form a reliable opinion.

4 [2020] EWHC 2129 QB

3   **Where the person gets lost in the process – some cases to consider**

Sadly, there is a significant minority of cases in which the assessment process can dominate to the detriment of the person being assessed. Here are two exemplar cases which do no credit to those in the statutory sector who are driving them.

EB was a young man who had complex Cerebral Palsy as a result of a complicated birth. He had attended specialist educational provision and residential schooling until adulthood. The support that he received from his father and step-mother was exemplary and second to none. They were his advocates with professionals and sought to empower him in decision-making at every turn. They subjugated their needs to ensure that he had the best possible quality of life. He was dependent for all care over a 24-hour period.

During his 20s, the family relocated to a different area of the UK. The statutory services (Local Authority and Clinical Commissioning Group) did not know (or engage well) with **EB** and his family. From the outset, they did not understand his brain injury and sought to deny him access to services that he had been entitled to and enjoyed for many years where he previously lived. The focus of the engagement by statutory services appeared to be one of minimising cost. Whilst **EB** had received a financial settlement because of clinical errors made during his birth, this was held on Trust and had been judiciously used to provide him with holidays and special therapy services that were not otherwise available, such as hydrotherapy. It is understood that the financial settlement had been approved by the Court on the basis that the statutory services would meet their obligations to **EB** and he would not be required to fund these out of his settlement.

However, when **EB** moved, the new local Clinical Commissioning Group and Social Services departments insisted on carrying out a comprehensive review, which included an assessment of his capacity to make decisions about his care. However, they failed to involve either **EB** or his family in their decision-making, refusing to accept existing, independent evidence that he did, in fact, have mental capacity to make such decisions. Appointments to visit him at home were made with short or no notice, no provision was made to attempt to communicate with **EB** on his level (he had profound communication difficulties) and both he and his family were railroaded into accepting care from non-specialist providers who were not trained in use of the specialist equipment that **EB** needed. Mistakes in the provision of his care occurred, and his family raised a series of safeguarding issues. **EB** became increasingly distressed, and there was a recurrence of challenging behaviour which had not been seen for many years. He began to refuse food as a means of communicating his distress. The family became labelled as "difficult". An impasse was reached. Communication broke down completely between the family and statutory services. The statutory services persisted with their approach to decide what to provide, and how to provide support and care services in **EB**'s best interests but did not seek the views of either **EB** or his family and their privately paid carers who knew him well.

EC was a young adult who had sustained a catastrophic ABI as a young teenager which had left him completely dependent for all his care needs. He was rehabilitated in hospital and specialist residential provision for some time before returning home to a tight-knit, loving and supportive family. **EC** attended specialist education provision for teenagers with special needs and was well assessed, understood and supported at the facility. The staff engaged with his family and communicated well throughout so that there was mutual respect and support.

When **EC** transitioned into adulthood, the Local Authority (LA) and CCG provided for him from Learning Disability services who lacked the specialist knowledge, skills or training to work with a person with an ABI. Services became critical of **EC**'s mother, as she frequently challenged their lack of appropriate provision for her son.

Matters came to a head when the authorities insisted that **EC** be moved away from home to a specialist brain injury residential unit to be assessed over a several-month period. **EC** had consistently stated his wish to remain at home and in his local community, where he had considerable family support and engaged well in activities. **EC**'s mother and family challenged the decision to move him, and the matter ended up in court. The authorities insisted that it was in **EC**'s *"best interests"* to be assessed at this unit, a tacit (although hidden) acknowledgement that they lacked the understanding of brain injury at the highest level of the CCG and LA.

Mother quite rightly pointed out that one cannot consider Best Interests decision-making without first having assessed **EC**'s capacity to make the decision. At this point, a Social Worker (who had never before met **EC**) visited him twice. Each appointment lasted no more than 15 minutes. The opinion expressed by the Social Worker was that he clearly lacked capacity. However, no attempt had been made to share the information relevant to the decision with **EC** or to consult those who knew and supported him how best to communicate with him. His Communication Passport was not referred to by the Social Worker, and her notes indicated that she had asked him closed questions on difficult concepts. She had not explained, for example, that he would be staying away from home for several months if he was placed at the specialist assessment unit. She did not appreciate that he had no understanding of the concept of "time".

Once again, mother challenged the assessment in terms of its validity. Once again, she was ignored. The CCG sent in a Clinical Psychologist who was trained and working in the Learning Disability specialty to assess **EC**'s wishes and feelings. The Psychologist similarly failed to use the Communication Passport and refused the mother or carers access to the sessions. Mother could see that **EC** was distressed and did not want to communicate with the Psychologist. The carers offered to help the Psychologist to understand **EC**'s communication, and the offer was rejected. The Psychologist insisted on being accompanied by a Physiotherapy technician who had never met **EC** before. Clearly, a skilled Speech and Language Therapist would have been a more appropriate choice in the circumstances.

In my opinion, these are two examples of a situation cited in published MCA literature with alarming frequency which illustrate how _not_ to assess capacity for making decisions around care needs in the absence of understanding of brain injury (Odumuyiwa et al., 2019).

Key
Learning
Points

How to ensure that the process is fair, robust and transparent:

- Those involved in assessing capacity where there is underlying brain injury MUST have specialist training and support or supervision in brain injury.
- The Code of Practice and NICE Guidance on Decision-Making and Mental Capacity must be followed if the assessment and outcome are to be valid.
- The person must sit at the centre of the assessment, their wishes, beliefs and feelings must be appropriately sought, acknowledged and included in any process where the outcome affects their life.
- The authorities must also consult the family and carers of the person being assessed to ensure that they have fully understood the person's needs for support to communicate and engage in the process.

4   Giving oral evidence in the Court of Protection

It is important to recognise that assessments that are undertaken to assist the Court in matters of mental capacity all have the potential to be provided as oral evidence before a Judge. Cases have been cited earlier in this chapter of Neuropsychologists in particular who have been instrumental in assisting the Court in matters of executive dysfunction in the context of decision-making. However, it is clear that other professionals, such as Consultant Psychiatrists, are similarly well positioned to assist the Court. Ruck-Keene et al. (2019) comment that"

> *Contested cases hinge on the "use or weigh" ability, Psychiatrists should be aware that good quality evidence on this ability is particularly pertinent in Court* (p. 70).

Here are some case presentations of giving oral evidence in the Court of Protection.

ED is a 65-year-old man with ARBD who found himself ordered to a specialist placement by the Courts and where he was subject to DoLS. He contested his DoLS on the basis that he did not need any help or support with activities of daily living, managing his money or taking his medication. His arguments were based on his views that he did not have brain damage and had no medical conditions which required medication. He was supported by an advocate and an adult daughter.

He lacked any insight or (intellectual) awareness of his brain injury or his needs. He was unable to lay down new memories, and although considerable work was undertaken to enable him to learn behavioural routines to support his memory difficulties, he failed to adapt in any way. Without 24-hour support in place, he would not have been able to meet his own needs.

On a previous occasion when he had been taken off a DoLS, **ED** had left the unit and engaged in binge drinking. He went missing for several days and was found by the Police with no money in a town some 40 miles away where he did not know anyone or have any form of shelter. He has since denied that this ever occurred.

ED's Social Worker was remarkably skilled and had patiently spent many hours with him explaining options, understanding his views and supporting him as far as possible. However, she clearly understood that he was presenting with a "*cloak of competence*", as he was verbally articulate and plausible but that this was only evident on superficial questioning. **ED**'s daughter expressed a similar view that her father would "*say one thing but do another*" and she remained concerned as to what might happen should the DoLS be lifted.

The Neuropsychologist was unable to assess him face-to-face because a lockdown was in place but was able to conduct a series of remote interviews both with **ED** and with significant others. It became clear early on in the assessment that **ED** had some awareness of his memory deficits, as he would become defensive if questioned closely about issues relating to his care and also his previous experiences when not under DoLS.

As matters progressed, the Court became most concerned about his capacity to self-administer medication and to make decisions about care and treatment. The Neuropsychologist was able to explain to the Court why the attempt to teach him to self-medicate had failed (which it did, with considerable risk to **ED**'s health, when he overdosed on an anti-convulsant tablet) and the role of frontal lobe paradox in his clinical presentation. Much of the questioning in Court indicated that many of those present had no grasp of this aspect of **ED**'s difficulties and were somewhat stuck on the "empowerment" agenda of seeking to enable him to achieve the greatest independence by not restricting his rights and freedoms. The Neuropsychologist was able to provide the Judge with a framework of understanding by linking the ARBD with real-life examples of how this impacting his decision-making, placing him at significant risk as a result.

EE was a young adult who had sustained a moderate traumatic brain injury as a 12-year-old. Her family had always insisted that her personality had changed as a result, but she had been lost to follow up between two different NHS Trusts. She had struggled at school and left without qualifications. Her relationships with her family had broken down, and she was raised by her maternal grandmother. Whilst still a teenager, she met a young man with whom she entered into an intimate, and somewhat violent, relationship which resulted in the birth of a child who was immediately placed on the Child Protection Register. One of the conditions placed upon her continuing to parent her son was that she ceased having contact with the father and ended the relationship on the grounds that he had been consistently violent towards her during the pregnancy. Social Services became aware that **EE** had maintained contact with the father and had met him in secret, taking the son along to meet him. The Court then placed both mother and baby in a specialist unit for 12 weeks, where the focus was on providing support in a competence-promoting way. However, whilst there she continued to have secret contact with the father and met him for sex. She became pregnant again but miscarried within a few weeks of confirmation of pregnancy.

The Court of Protection were involved in terms of needing to assess her mental capacity to make decisions around keeping her child safe from harm. The Neuropsychologist was

instructed to assist the Court and was able to provide unequiv-
ocal evidence of neurocognitive impairment such that the
diagnostic test of the MCA was satisfied. It became clear from
interviews, comprehensive records and assessment that **EE** was
unable to put any knowledge into practice in terms of _using_ the
information she had acquired at the mother-and-baby unit.
If interviewed, she was well able to explain what she should
do. She was aware of the risks posed by the father of her son
but was unable to use that information to prevent her having
contact which risked the child being removed from her care.
During oral evidence to the Court, the Neuropsychologist was
asked how EE differed from many other mothers who come
through the Family Law Courts with similar parenting difficulties. This provided an opportunity to place the traumatic brain
injury at the centre of all considerations of mother's abilities.

Key	Pointers for giving oral evidence:
Learning	• Be clear how the brain injury is central to understanding the person's difficulties.
Points	• Be clear that the Code of Practice and all relevant guidance was followed in terms of due process and weight given to key matters.
	• Be transparent in describing what information was used to inform the expert opinion in relation to mental capacity.
	• Be clear about what support the person might need going forward in terms of their rights and freedoms when balanced against safety considerations.

5 *Best Interests impasse (Chapter 15 Code of Practice)*

•   _Between clinicians and family_

EF was an elderly man who had sustained an acquired
brain injury as a result of a clinically negligent act whilst in
hospital. A doctor had removed a central line incorrectly

which had caused an explosion of bubbles of oxygen throughout his brain, described by the neuroradiologist as having the effect of fireworks going off in his brain.

He was the head of a strong and tightly-knit family who were suspicious of any treatment offered and extremely protective of him. He was discharged home with an experienced brain injury case manager and a full 24-hour care and rehabilitation package. From the outset, despite considerable efforts to engage with the EF 's adult daughters, clinicians and care staff were treated with contempt. Every clinical decision was questioned, and on more than one occasion threats were made to staff by members of the family.

One such issue which arose was the decision by the clinical team to apply for a DoLS in order to have an anti-tamper lap-belt fitted to EF 's wheelchair to stop him trying to stand up. He was unaware that he could no longer stand unaided or walk as a result of his brain injury and would frequently place himself and care staff at risk by impulsively trying to stand. Attempts to intervene frequently resulted in an escalation of his behaviour to the point where he would punch staff. At the Best Interests Decision meeting to consider the special lap-belt as an option, his family were angry and refused to consider this, describing it in pejorative terms and seeing it only as a restriction. An impasse was reached, with the family becoming increasingly aggressive. The meeting was adjourned to allow time and space to reflect on the issues.

Considerable efforts were then expended in listening to the family's concerns and explaining the clinical risks of not providing the lap-belt. The family were encouraged to take their time in researching the issues and options for themselves and communication was maintained between a nominated family member and the case manager. The family came to realise that the proposed lap-belt was the least restrictive option available to keep EF safe, and they came on board with the decision which was then collectively made in his best interests. If this collaborative conclusion had not been reached, then there was the possibility of mediation or of applying the Court of Protection, but at that point it is likely that relationships would have broken down around EF which would have been detrimental to his care.

• _Between past and present wishes of same person_

EG was a transgender person who was mid-transition from male to female. EG had a long history of bipolar disorder, and on one occasion when they had been sectioned under the Mental Health Act, had received an overdose of Lithium in error, resulting in an ABI. EG 's mental health remained unstable, and they struggled to make any decisions regarding daily life. EG would give away money to strangers; make unfounded allegations about care staff members, leading to difficulties recruiting and retaining support staff; and express violent rages, during which they would self-harm. Staff were briefed not to accept any gifts from EG in case they were misinterpreted by them, but when this occurred, EG would become distressed, as they thought it meant that staff did not like them, and allegations would ensue.

The Neuropsychologist was asked to assess EG 's testamentary capacity because they expressed the desire the change their Will on a weekly basis. Whenever EG met a new person in their life, they would begin to buy them gifts and then promise to leave them a legacy in their Will. EG had a Court Appointed Deputy who carefully balanced EG 's rights to have a degree of financial freedom with the need to prevent them from financial exploitation.

During the capacity assessment, it became clear that EG could not remember all of their previous wishes in terms of legacies and, over repeated appointments, would express contrary views and plans. AsRuck-Keene et al. (2017) put it:

> Which version of their autonomy should we seek to honour? . . . . What would be the right thing to do in this situation? Would it be to exercise her precedent autonomy or her current wishes and feelings? (pp. 133–134).

It could be argued that there is no "psychological continuity" (Dresser, 1995, p. 33) between the pre- and post- brain injury **EG**, and that essentially they are different people, and as such the most recent wishes should be upheld, particularly if **EG** cannot recall their previous position and will never regain mental capacity.

The assessment concluded that **EG** lacked the mental capacity to make a valid Will and continued to need assistance with managing property and affairs. A Statutory Will was applied for.

Key Learning Points	• Always keep clear lines of communication open to avoid, if possible, an impasse in decision-making.
	• If possible and practicable, postpone the best interests' decision for a short period to allow the parties time to do their own research, to reflect and to consider.
	• Where there is an impasse between previously expressed wishes and currently expressed wishes, care needs to be taken as to how much weight to apply to each, based on individual circumstances.

Reflections of a professional

Dr Peter Marshall – Consultant Neuropsychiatrist

This excellent chapter is a must-read for professionals involved in MCA assessments of individuals with ABI. Assessing Mental Capacity in individuals with ABI can be complicated, and the examples clearly highlight this.

The general awareness within services supporting individuals with ABI, can be limited, in relation to the frequency of OPD (also known as dysexecutive syndrome) and its presence (even if there is a lack of evidence of frontal lobe involvement at the time of injury) and its impact on MCA assessments. Lack of awareness of the frontal lobe paradox does result in disagreements around capacity, and these cases do end up in Court – often a protracted and distressing process for the individual which can impact on the treatment plan. Increased understanding of this issue may reduce Court of Protection applications and the stress this causes to an individual.

Adoption of the key learning points within this chapter, such as gaining collateral information (highlighting discrepancies between what an individual says and does), will be a move in the right direction and will make a difference to the validity of MCA assessments of individuals with the frontal lobe paradox.

Dr Mark Holloway – Specialist Social Worker

There is a significant difference between intellectual awareness and insight. I have witnessed people being assumed to have insight because:

- A woman knew her name and where she was;
- A man knew he had experienced a brain injury; and
- A man, in conversation with a social worker, acknowledged he had a brain injury and that he struggled with his memory.

The capacity for a brain injured person to define their difficulty and state what strategy is required to compensate for this does not, in and of itself, mean that they have developed sufficient awareness of their difficulties to actually act in accordance with this knowledge. Intellectual awareness is not insight, and, for those who are brain injury unaware (or who do not seek third-party corroborative evidence) the brain-injured person can be very plausible.

An overly simplistic application of the social model of disability frequently fails brain-injured people who lack insight as there is no self-identification of disability, making decisions and choices are executive functions that can be impaired (sometimes severely without diminution of intelligence) and the act of the brain-injured party intellectually recognising and discussing their needs does not equate to having insight and being able to respond to them. The skill of working with such individuals is to incorporate the values and of the social model, issues of choice, empowerment, partnership and collaboration (Trevillion, 2007), but to do so in the context of the brain injury and its impact upon functioning, especially when insight is a confounding issue.

One of the functional issues we see, outside of externally generated and extrinsically governed structures, is that many of our people fail to generate ideas when required or fail to generate more than one idea. I think that this may be the issue with the "Good in Theory, Poor in Practice" that we see. This is also why, in assessments, when the assessor generates the ideas, people appear more competent. In real-world settings, where we need to respond to feedback from the environment and adjust our actions and behaviour in real time, such people perform so badly. Difficulties with problem solving can have, as their root, difficulties with idea generation. When this is the case, problem-solving strategies cannot simply be applied by the brain-injured party, as the options to weigh up and decide between cannot be generated in the first place. In this instance, a difficulty with idea generation can become a significant handicap to an individual, particularly when dealing with novel situations, and this has an impact upon functional independence and employability. Experience shows that difficulties with idea generation and initiation are often misattributed to issues of motivation (notwithstanding the fact that difficulties with poor idea generation and the associated task failure experienced may be demotivating per se). A lack of insight into this difficulty will compound the problems faced by the brain injured party as all "blame" for failure and difficulty is externalised, and so learning opportunities are limited. A behavioural response simply to reject ideas provided by others is further disabling for those who cannot idea generate.

References & weblinks

Cameron, E. & Codling, J. (in press) Myth Buster: Demystifying the terms decisional/executive capacity and executive functioning/dysfunction in the context of the Mental Capacity Act (2005).

Decision-Making and Mental Capacity. (2018) NICE. www.nice.org.uk/guidance/ng108/resources/decisionmaking-and-mental-capacity-pdf-66141544670917

Dresser, R. (1995) Dworkin on dementia: Elegant theory, questionable policy. *The Hastings Centre Report, 25* (6).

George, M. & Gilbert, S. (2018) Mental Capacity Act (2005) assessments: Why everyone needs to know about the frontal lobe paradox. *The Neuropsychologist, 5*, pp. 59–66.

Knight, C.; Alderman, N. & Burgess, P. W. (2002) Development of a simplified version of the multiple errands test for use in hospital settings. *Neuropsychological Rehabilitation, 12* (3), pp. 231–255. DOI:10.1080/09602010244000039

Marsh, H. (2017) *Admissions: A life in brain surgery*. Orion Books (London)

McMillan, T. & Wood, R. (2017) *Neurobehavioural disability and social handicap following traumatic brain injury* (Second edition). Abingdon, UK: Routledge.

Mental Capacity Act Code of Practice. (2007) www.gov.uk/government/publications/mental-capacity-act-code-of-practice

Moore, S.; Wotus, R.; Norman, A.; Holloway, M. & Dean, J. (2019) Behind the cloak of competence: Brain injury and mental capacity legislation. *The Journal of Adult Protection, 21* (4), pp. 201–218.

Odumuyiwa, T.; Kennedy, M.; Norman, A.; Holloway, M.; Suffield, F.; Forrest, H. & Dicks, H. (2019) Improving access to social care services following acquired brain injury: A needs analysis. *Journal of Long Term Care*, pp. 164–175.

Owen, G.; Freyenhagen, F. & Martin, W. (2019) Assessing decision-making capacity after brain injury: A phenomenological approach. *Philosophy, Psychiatry & Psychology, 25* (1), pp. 1–19.

Ruck-Keene, A.; Cooper, R. & Hobbs, T. (2017) When past and present wishes collides: The theory, the practice and the future. www.mentalcapacitylawandpolicy.org.uk/wp-content/uploads/2017/11/When-wishes-and-feelings-collide.pdf

Ruck-Keene, A,; Kane, N. B.; Kim, S. Y. H. & Owen, G. S. (2019) Taking capacity seriously? Ten years of mental capacity disputes before England's Court of Protection. *International Journal of Law and Psychiatry, 62*, pp.56-76

Shallice, T. & Burgess, P. W. (1991) Deficits in strategy application following frontal lobe damage in man. *Brain, 114*, pp. 727–741.

Teuber, H. L. (1964) The riddle of the frontal lobe function in man. In J. M. Warren & K. Akert (eds.) *The frontal granular cortex and behaviour* (pp. 410–458). New York: McGraw-Hill.

Trevillion, S. (2007) Critical commentary: Health, disability and social work: New directions in social work research. *British Journal of Social Work, 37*, pp. 937–946.

UKABIF Open Letter. (6th March 2019) Mental Capacity Act code of practice: Call for evidence.

Wood, R. L. & Bigler, E. (2017) Problems assessing executive dysfunction in neurobehavioural disability. Chapter 7 in T. M. McMillan & R. L. Wood (eds.) *Neurobehavioural disability and social handicap following traumatic brain injury* (Second edition). Abingdon, UK: Routledge.

www.bps.org.uk/blogs/guest/parliament-and-%E2%80%98frontal-lobe-paradox%E2%80%99

Chapter 6

Common assessments of mental capacity – cases to consider

1 Discharge Destination

There are two interesting cases reported which provide some guidance as to the Court of Protection's approach to the issues of discharge and decisions around care.

The first, reported in 2013[1], established the key components of an assessment that are required when assessing an individual's ability to make decisions about where they will live next, whether on discharge from hospital or moving on to stepped down supported care.

a) The two (or more) options for living. This must include the type and nature of the living option, such as whether it amounts to supported living or not, and if so, in what way P will be supported. P must also understand what sort of property it is and the facilities that would be available to them there.

b) Broad information about the area. This would cover the notional 'sort' of area in which the property is located and any known specific risks of living in that area beyond the usual risks faced by people living in any other given area.

c) The difference between living somewhere and just visiting it. Pictorial methods of conducting this assessment may be useful. This could include a discussion of what it means to

1 [2013] EWHC 3230 (Fam)

DOI: 10.4324/9781003205210-6

sleep somewhere and an understanding of the days of the week (and so on).

d)   The activities that P would be able to do if they lived in each place.

e)   Whether and how P would be able to see friends and family if they lived in each place.

f)   The payment of rent and bills. This is not required to be understood in any detail beyond the fact that there will have to be a payment made on their behalf.

g)   Any rules of compliance and/or the general obligations of a tenancy. The rules are not required to be known in any great detail by P, but a basic understanding of the fact that there are restrictions, and the areas in which they would operate, will be necessary.

h)   Who they would be living with at each placement.

i)   The sort of care they would receive in each placement.

j)   The risk that a family member or other contact may not wish to see P should they choose a particular placement against their family's wishes.

The following information is _not_ relevant to a decision as to capacity concerning residence arrangements:

a)   The cost of the placement and/or the value of money. The details of the precise financial arrangements are not important to the question of capacity beyond a basic understanding of whether payment is required.

b)   The legal nature of the tenancy agreement or licence.

c)   The consequences on the nature of the relationship of P with a contact or family member in the long term (10 to 20 years) should the former choose to live independently.

The following is relevant information to an assessment of whether P has capacity to decide their own care:

a)   What areas P needs support with;

b)   What sort of support they need;

c)   Who will provide such support;

d)   What would happen without support, or if support was refused; and

e) That carers may not always treat the person being cared for properly, and the possibility and mechanics of making a complaint if they are not happy.

The following are <u>not</u> relevant to an assessment of capacity as to care:

a) How care is funded.
b) How overarching arrangements for monitoring and appointing care staff work.

The second case is more recent, from 2021,[2] and concerns the case of an individual refusing to be discharged from hospital to a place chosen by others, in his best interests. The individual in this case was considered to:

> *Require support with the following areas of his care: medication administration and management; mental health/behaviour management and potential aggression; physical health management regarding diabetes, refusal to attend medical assessments/have health checks completed; self-care prompts in relation to hygiene and dressing; shopping; housekeeping; social inclusion and activities; community access; continued finance management. . . . X could pose a risk to himself and potentially others if he did not receive care support as outlined above* (paragraph 40).

The judge in this case set out what he considered to be the key issues to resolve the matter of disputed discharge:

> i) *Is it in X's best interests for him to leave X Hospital? There is a broad consensus as to the answer to this question, but I consider that it ought nonetheless to be asked and answered given X's clear views/opposition;*
> ii) *Which alternative residential care establishment would best meet X's needs? Is this likely to be X House? Or another resource in Town A or elsewhere? It was previously said that a resource called XY in Town A may be a suitable placement, but no places were available at the date of the previous hearing. The LA and the CCG have*

    confirmed that if they become aware of a vacancy at this placement
    prior to the final hearing the litigation friend would be notified.
  iii) *What steps can/should be taken to prepare X for any move?*
  iv) *How, physically and emotionally, can X be moved in a way which*
     best meets his needs, fulfils his best interests and offers the least
     restrictions?
   v) *If he is to move, when and in what circumstances should the deci-*
    sion be communicated to him?
  vi) *How should it be communicated to him, and what support should*
    be offered to him at that time? . . .
 viii) *Who should be involved in preparing X for any move and for*
    effecting any move?
  ix) *What role will the family play in that endeavour?*
   x) *What are X's views about the proposals? (paragraph 48)*

With this legal framework in view, here are some cases to consider.

    FA was a 60-year-old woman who had sustained a severe trau-
matic brain injury as a result of a fall downstairs at home whilst
intoxicated. She sustained significant facial and bony injuries
within the skull as well as significant brain bleeding which raised
the pressure inside her head. Once her injuries settled, she was able
to be transferred to a post-acute neurorehabilitation where she
was treated by neuro-specialists. As she made progress week-on-
week with her rehabilitation goals, discussions were started with
FA, her family and her social worker regarding her discharge destination and her care and support needs post-discharge. Clinically,
she was assessed as having gross cognitive impairment including
attention and memory deficits, as well as executive impairments
in terms of cognitive flexibility, problem-solving, perspective taking, abstract and consequential reasoning. However, **FA** did not
have any language impairments and was able to converse fluently.
She was pleasant and engaging with patients and staff alike but
fatigued extremely easily because of significant slowing in her
ability to process information as a result of her brain injury. She
had a complete lack of insight into her injury and its effects and
although she demonstrated intellectual awareness, (e.g., she knew
that she had sustained a brain injury) she was not able to use this
information within her decision-making.

FA considered herself ready for discharge home and did not need any support. She was unable to apply her knowledge of the benefits to herself of the structure and support of the ward environment with what needs she may have when home. She had previously lived alone and independently and felt, without any direct evidence, that she could do so successfully on discharge.

Work was done with **FA** to help her to increase her emergent awareness (where intellectual awareness combines with personal experience to result in a degree of insight). She was supported to make connections between her needs for support on the ward to how this might translate to need for support at home, but she remained singularly unable to do so. Like many people who have had a brain injury, she harboured the belief that once she was home, everything would return to "normal" (that is, her pre-injury level of functioning). With the support of her family, she was able to try a brief period of home leave which proved instructive to both her and the clinical team as to her ongoing needs.

FB was a 50-year-old man who had fallen down stairs whilst moving furniture into a new home. He sustained a severe traumatic brain injury which required a lengthy stay in hospital, moving from acute care to inpatient neurorehabilitation prior to discharge. His cognitive impairment was such that he had no recollection of the period leading up to his house move (retrograde amnesia) and believed he still lived at a former address. He was able to recall his family, but would mix up his own life facts with those of other family members. He was physically unimpaired and was independently mobile on the ward. He was assessed as having significant cognitive (attention, memory, language) difficulties but was fluent in his conversation. At face value, he appeared unimpaired, but when attempts were made to engage him in anything other than brief conversational small talk, it would become apparent that he struggled to both understand what others were saying and to express what he wanted to say coherently.

As a complicating factor, during his stay on the ward, it became apparent that his marital relationship was not robust and had been at the point of breakdown at the time of injury. **FB**, however, had no recollection of this. This meant that preparations for discharge were complex, as his wife did not want him discharged to their home, but he could not understand why this was not possible. The clinical team worked hard with **FB** and his social worker to consider all possible discharge options and to assess his ability to make a decision in respect of what support he might need. This included considering all options and involving his wider family. He was eventually able to be discharged to a stepped-down placement to the area where his biological family lived and where he had lifelong friends. This enabled him to prepare for a new, post-injury independence but one in which his needs for care and support could be met from a wide range of sources in order to maximise his well-being and sense of belonging.

FC was a non-UK national who was on a working visa when she was struck by a bus whilst crossing the road in the town where she worked. She sustained a severe traumatic brain injury as a result and was in hospital for many months for both acute care and neurorehabilitation. During the period of recovery and treatment, it emerged that there was a significant rift and mutual mistrust between her partner (with whom she lived for part of each week) and her daughter, who remained living in their country of origin. Each made contact with the professionals concerned with **FC**'s care to register complaints concerning the financial motivations of the other. **FC** was not aware of this undercurrent for several months.

As **FC** progressed with her neurorehabilitation, it became necessary to carry out a mental capacity assessment of her ability to decide where she wished to live upon discharge. Whilst she had been in hospital, her daughter had travelled to the UK and had emptied **FC**'s apartment and given notice on her tenancy on her behalf, on the advice of the doctors who first treated **FC** and did not expect her to survive. This meant that **FC** could no longer return home. The point was moot, however, as she lacked insight into her care and support needs and had a completely unrealistic understanding of her retained abilities.

The options for residence after discharge became binary. **FC** could either move in with her partner full-time, even though they had never lived together fully before and though he lived several hours away from her friends and former workplace. Moreover, her partner worked full-time, which meant that he would be unable to provide support during work hours. Both **FC** and her partner were keen for this option. The alternative option was that **FC**'s Social Worker would find her a new place to live in the area where she lived prior to her injury and had friends who could support her. Whilst all of the preparation work was being undertaken in order to support **FC** to make a decision, the local Safeguarding team became involved following a referral for financial exploitation of **FC** by her partner. This meant that his home could no longer be considered as a potential discharge destination whilst the investigation was underway. **FC** was considered to be financially vulnerable, and control of her finances came under the Court of Protection from that point.

The outcome was that **FC** was involved in selecting a suitable temporary placement in a local rehabilitation facility where she would have a flat of her own but where there would be 24-hour provision of care and support staff. This would enable **FC** to maximise her potential for independent living in the local community prior to any decision regarding her longer-term living arrangements. The discharge took place as planned without further difficulty.

Key
Learning
Points

- All assessments of capacity to decide discharge destination must take into account a wide range of factors:

  o   The structured environment of a ward or care placement provides significant (but hidden) support in terms of the routine and prompting that is provided. Consider how the person would cope without this.

o   Consider all relevant family factors – are the relationships robust enough to withstand the support demands? Is what the family saying they can provide realistic and sustainable in terms of support? Are the family putting pressure on the person to live in a particular place?

o   Does the person have more than just intellectual awareness of their impairments and difficulties? Do they really understand what their needs are and how they might be met when they leave?

o   Is a period of home leave possible or practicable?

o   Is there a plan in place for if the discharge arrangement fails?

2   Property and Affairs (finances)

The Act provides that capacity is time-specific and decision-specific, and must be assessed in relation to each decision, at the time that decision needs to be made. However, the Code of Practice suggests that where the impairment or disturbance is ongoing or long-term, this may be relevant to an assessment of the person's capacity to manage their property and affairs more generally. This approach was recognised by the Court of Protection, where

> The general concept of managing affairs is an ongoing act and, therefore, quite unlike the specific act of making a will or making an enduring power of attorney. The management of affairs related to a continuous state of affairs whose demands may be unpredictable and may occasionally be urgent.[3]

3 [2012] EWHC 2400 (COP) paragraph 41

In any assessment of an individual's ability to manage their finances and affairs, the following areas must be considered:

- The extent of the person's property and affairs, which would include an examination of:

  - Income and capital (including savings and the value of the home), expenditure, and liabilities;
  - Financial needs and responsibilities;
  - Whether there are likely to be any changes in the person's financial circumstances in the foreseeable future;
  - The skill, specialised knowledge and time it takes to manage the affairs properly and whether the impairment of, or disturbance in the functioning of, the person's mind or brain is affecting the management of the assets; and
  - Whether the person would be likely to seek, understand and act on appropriate advice where needed in view of the complexity of the affairs.

- *Personal information:*

  - Age,
  - Life expectancy,
  - Past medical history,
  - Prospects of recovery or deterioration,
  - The extent to which capacity could fluctuate,
  - The condition in which the person lives,
  - Family background and family and social responsibilities,
  - Any cultural, ethnic or religious considerations, and
  - The degree of support the person receives (or could expect to receive) from others.

- *A person's vulnerability:*

  - Could an inability to manage the property and affairs lead to the person making rash or irresponsible decisions?
  - Could an inability to manage lead to exploitation by others – perhaps even by family members?
  - Could an inability to manage lead to the position of other people being compromised or jeopardised?

FD was a young adult male who had sustained a severe brain injury as a result of accidentally ingesting methadone as a young child. He had been awarded a substantial financial settlement as a result, which had been kept in Trust until he reached adulthood. One of the Trustees was a family member who exerted significant and substantial influence over **FD** in all matters. **FD** had complained to many clinicians and support workers over several years that he was desperate to get out from under the control of this relative but was afraid of repercussions. A formal assessment upon his reaching 18 had concluded that he lacked the capacity to manage his financial affairs, and the Court of Protection had appointed Joint Deputies, one of whom was a Solicitor and the other the relative who exerted control over **FD**.

FD had been assessed as having significant cognitive impairment and had been shown to be highly suggestible, meaning that he was susceptible to influence. **FD** requested a repeat assessment of his capacity to manage his affairs. The Deputies gave joint instruction as to the assessment, who was to be consulted and how and what specific questions were to be answered by the assessment. **FD** presented as highly suspicious during the assessment and the impression was formed that he had been coached in what to say. He had some factual information learned by rote, but even then, there had been significant omissions in the information he was able to understand and recall around his finances over a series of appointments. He held fixed views and beliefs about his finances which did not appear to be his own views but those of his relative (and Deputy). For example, he was rigid in his belief that his other Deputy (Solicitor) had stolen from him since being appointed, despite there being no evidence, even following an investigation by the Office of the Public Guardian prompted by his relative. He consistently expressed the opinion that, "*I know what I have been told*" (referring to his relative).

The outcome of the assessment was that **FD** continued to lack the capacity to manage his finances and affairs and that he needed to be provided with independent advice about his finances because of his suggestibility.

FE was a young man who had sustained a traumatic brain injury in a road traffic collision as a teenager. He presented as

verbally plausible with little cognitive impairment, whereas
in reality he had been diagnosed with OPD as a result of his
brain injury. He initially came across as charming and engaging, but this could change in an instant to verbal and physical
aggression which placed him, and those around him at significant risk of injury. Generally, his behaviour was impulsive. He
would take drugs if offered any, drink to excess and start fights,
all of which resulted in him being banned from many pubs in
his local area. The police were also familiar with him and his
injury, and would frequently pick him up and take him home
to his parents rather than place him in the cells.

He eventually moved into his own house, bought on his
behalf by a Court-appointed Deputy for Property and Affairs.
All of his outgoing bills were paid directly by his Deputy. He
was provided with small amounts of money each week for living expenses, but he frequently spent this and borrowed more,
resulting in regular and sometimes abusive calls to his Deputy.

FE was firmly of the view that he was able to manage his
own finances and he resented having to ask his Deputy for
money. A repeat assessment was requested. **FE** presented for
assessment expressing the view that if it did not result in him
obtaining access to his finances it was a waste of his time. He
was unable to understand what monies were required to live
from week to week in his own accommodation, despite this
information being provided to him regularly by his Deputy in
both verbal and written form. **FE** was unable to recall how he
spent the money he was able to control and became demanding
of monies to buy equipment to set himself up in a business,
despite him having no training, experience or explicit business
planning for the venture. He held the view that his Deputy
was preventing him from living his "*best life*" which he would
be able to achieve without any help or support. This view ran
contrary to the evidence of his financial vulnerability and past
behaviours. A further concern was that the Deputy had had to
contact the Local Authority Safeguarding team when it came
to light that **FE** had been befriended by local drug dealers
who may have been trying to use his house as base from which
to operate. With regard to the re-assessment of capacity, the

decision was taken to register the outcome with the Court of Protection along with concerns regarding FE's susceptibility to influence. The relative of FE who served as a Deputy threatened to resign their position unless he was found to have capacity to manage his own affairs and to sue the professional who carried out the assessment. The matter continued.

FF was a young man who had a diagnosis of High-Functioning Autism (ASD) who had been attacked by a group of young males in the park near his home. In his attempt to escape, **FF** jumped off a low bridge but sustained a permanent spinal injury which was life-changing.

FF had been awarded a financial settlement as a result of his injuries, but there was concern expressed by his family and his solicitor that he may not have the mental capacity to manage his finances. The concern was based on numerous examples of him not being able to understand the value of money, of giving money away to strangers with no expectation of it being repaid and of him spending whatever money he had in his possession on others in order to gain their approbation or affection.

In this case, it was encouraging to learn the extent to which the family had sought to support **FF** in financial matters. He had a bank card and was able to recall his PIN, but was always accompanied by a close family member who provided support for him to withdraw money for himself, given the many previous experiences of him being financially exploited.

His father would go through weekly bank statements with **FF** to track spending and help **FF** to make plans for the week ahead, even though these were rarely stuck to by **FF**. The nature of family support was competence-promoting but even with this in place, it became clear that **FF** was extremely vulnerable.

A brief neurocognitive assessment examined **FF**'s abilities to use or weigh up financial information in a decision-making process and he performed at an extremely impaired level; specifically, in the bottom 2% of his peers within the general population. Essentially, **FF** lacked the mental flexibility that is required to support financial decision-making. An application was made to the Court of Protection to appoint a Deputy but

to maintain the support of the family in maximising his financial decision-making at every opportunity even within these
parameters.

Key Learning Points	• Individuals can appear competent but still be vulnerable to the influence of others. This susceptibility to influence can lead to them making (or attempting to make) decisions which are detrimental to their own well-being.
	• It is vital to consider that even when a person is of the view that they do not require support with their finances, any assessment must consider their vulnerabilities if they come under the auspices of the Mental Capacity Act.
	• Even when a person is deemed to lack capacity to manage their finances, it is important to continue to empower them towards the greatest level of autonomy that they can achieve whilst remaining financially safe.

3   Marry/pre-nuptial agreement/engage in sex/sex workers

The legal test for capacity to **marry** is straightforward and was
established by Munby J:[4]

> There are thus, in essence, two aspects to the inquiry whether
> someone has capacity to marry. (1) Does he or she understand the
> nature of the marriage contract? (2) Does he or she understand the
> duties and responsibilities that normally attach to marriage? . . .
>   The duties and responsibilities that normally attach to marriage
> can be summarised as follows: Marriage, whether civil or religious,
> is a contract, formally entered into. It confers on the parties the
> status of husband and wife, the essence of the contract being an

4 [2004] EWHC 2808 (Fam)Paragraph 141

> *agreement between a man and a woman to live together, and to love one another as husband and wife, to the exclusion of all others. It creates a relationship of mutual and reciprocal obligations, typically involving the sharing of a common home and a common domestic life and the right to enjoy each other's society, comfort and assistance.*

More recently, the specific issue of capacity to marry for a person with a brain injury was considered[5] and the judge, Mostyn J, considered that the second limb, namely that, "*the essence of marriage is for two people to live together and love one another*", does not hold in modern society.

It is understood that the legal test to enter into a **pre-nuptial agreement**, is that the individual needs to understand the specific contract at the specific point in time. The law requires that the person must have intended to enter in to such a contract that is legally binding. Francis J expressed the view that,

> *It is clear, at least on the present state of the law, that full and frank financial disclosure is regarded as one of the key building blocks of a successful prenuptial agreement.*[6]

FG was a man who had sustained a traumatic brain injury as a young adult. He had married his first girlfriend post-injury after only being together a matter of weeks and against the explicit wishes and advice of his family. The marriage lasted for four days, and there were serious implications for financial remedy given that **FG** had been in receipt of a substantial financial settlement in connection with his personal injury. The matter was concluded at the time on the basis that he lacked the mental capacity to be involved in the financial implications of the divorce proceedings.

Several years later, **FG** met and established a new relationship. They settled down together and, after a significant period of time, decided that they wished to marry. **FG**'s Court-Appointed Deputy made it clear that it needed to be established that he had both capacity to enter into a pre-nuptial agreement and to marry.

An assessment took place of **FG**, with his consent and understanding. It was established that the idea of a pre-nuptial agreement was his, and he believed that this would protect his money in the unforeseen event of a marital breakdown. The assessment took place over several appointments to ensure that **FG** had all of the information that he needed to make the decision and that he had an opportunity to consider matters appropriately. He was provided with a draft agreement to look over. He gave his reasoning for wishing the pre-nuptial agreement as "*if the marriage breaks down it's about protecting my house . . . I can't be taken to the cleaners like with my first wife*". **FG** was specifically questioned in relation to his understanding of a pre-nuptial agreement, his recollection of the details of the draft pre-nuptial agreement and its meaning. **FG** also confirmed that he would "*need to write a will afterwards which I'm going to do*".

FG was asked about the various aspects of the pre-nuptial agreement, and he volunteered information at each stage without requiring prompting. He was fully aware of the different amounts of money that he would be prepared to pay to his future wife should the marriage break down, dependent upon how long the marriage has lasted up to a maximum amount. He was similarly aware that any debts which may be in place at the point of marriage breakdown would be attributed to the individual who had accrued such debts.

FG was also asked about his understanding of the pre-nuptial agreement from different perspectives and to consider the implications of it being invoked. He was clear that he wished to marry his girlfriend, that the wedding was planned and would go ahead and that he fully expected the marriage to last for life. He was also aware that his finances needed to be protected and that his future wife was fully aware of the implications of the same and that she wished to enter into a pre-nuptial agreement fully and fairly. He clearly demonstrated his ability to communicate his decision regarding the pre-nuptial agreement throughout the interviews. The view was taken that, on balance, **FG** retained the capacity to enter into a pre-nuptial contract.

With respect to **capacity to marry**, **FG** was asked about the details of the planned marriage, and he was able to recall the date, the venue, the number of guests invited to the day reception and in the evening as well as progress with arrangements for the same. **FG** retains his personal view of marriage as one of faithfulness and love and *"to be there when times are hard even when arguing"*. **FG** was asked once again about the difference between co-habiting and marriage and continued in his view that there is a closeness in marriage which is not present when *"just living together"*. When asked about his motivations for marrying his girlfriend, he confirmed that he wishes to have a *"wife for life"* and is looking forward to calling her Mrs **FG**.

Time was taken to explore expectations of marriage on the part of **FG**, he had a clear understanding of their individual roles and responsibilities within the relationship and it was clear that faithfulness is a requirement which is his choice and aspiration. He was insightful into the fact that there may currently be an uneven distribution of the domestic workload and that his partner frequently voices her concerns about the same but that this does not affect the stability of the relationship at present or going into the proposed nuptials.

FG was clear that marrying his girlfriend is his choice and he considered that, although he was *"gullible before, . . . I have learned so much"*. **FG** formed the view that following his brain injury he had come to appreciate life more and that his values had changed. He was clear that he loved his girlfriend in a deeper way than the emotions he expressed in relation to his first wife, which he categorised as *"lust"*.

FG confirmed that he and his partner did argue but that he continued to diffuse their arguments wherever possible by injecting humour and offering to make cups of tea. **FG** did, on the balance of probabilities, retain sufficient decision-making capacity to enter into the proposed marriage. His understanding of the decision to marry was clear, and his ability to recall the key information relating to entering into marriage and being married was similarly transparent and consistent. **FG** was able to sufficiently weigh and balance the considerations required to enter into a marital undertaking, and he was clearly able to communicate his wishes. He appeared to have benefitted from his experiences and was realistic about his future.

The legal test for **capacity to decide to have sex** has formed over time.

> *The approach taken in the line of first instance decisions . . . in regarding the test for capacity to consent to sexual relationships as being general and issue specific, rather than person or event specific, represents the correct approach within the terms of the MCA 2005.*[7]
>
> *It is an assessment of whether the person being assessed has the ability to understand those matters when explained to him or her and to retain the information for a period of time and to use or weigh it in deciding whether or not to consent to sexual relations.*[8]

The court most recently considered the issue of capacity to consent to sexual relations. Lord Justice Baker held that *"the "relevant information" must be tailored to the facts of the case"*.[9] This is a significant case which substantially updates the previous guidance on this issue. Lord Justice Baker concluded that there was a need to distinguish two separate questions:

(1) Whether someone has the capacity to consent to sexual relations, and
(2) Whether someone has the ability to choose whether or not to engage in sexual activity.

Lord Justice Baker went on to clarify the distinction:

> *The "information relevant to the decision" inevitably includes the fact that any person with whom P engages in sexual activity must be able to consent to such activity and does in fact consent to it. Sexual relations between human beings are mutually consensual. It is one of the many features that makes us unique. A person who does not understand that sexual relations must only take place when, and only for as long as, the other person is consenting*

7 [2014] EWCA Civ 37 paragraph 79
8 [2019] EWCA Civ 913 paragraph 57
9 [2020] EWCA Civ 735 paragraph 42

is unable to understand a fundamental part of the information relevant to the decision whether or not to engage in such relations (paragraph 94).

He reiterated that: "*the information which a capacitous individual must take into account in deciding whether to engage in sexual relations includes whether or not the other person is consenting*" (paragraph 99).

Lord Justice Baker went on to set out a list of information which may be relevant to the decision to engage in sexual relations:

In summary, when considering whether, as a result of an impairment of, or disturbance in the functioning of, the mind or brain, a person is unable to understand, retain, or use or weigh information relevant to a decision whether to engage in sexual relations, the information relevant to the decision may include the following:

(a) *the sexual nature and character of the act of sexual intercourse, including the mechanics of the act;*

(b) *the fact that the other person must have the capacity to consent to the sexual activity and must in fact consent before and throughout the sexual activity;*

(c) *the fact that P can say yes or no to having sexual relations and is able to decide whether to give or withhold consent;*

(d) *that a reasonably foreseeable consequence of sexual intercourse between a man and woman is that the woman will become pregnant;*

(e) *that there are health risks involved, particularly the acquisition of sexually transmitted and transmissible infections, and that the risk of sexually transmitted infection can be reduced by the taking of precautions such as the use of a condom.*

FH is a young woman who sustained an acquired brain injury in early childhood through a malignant brain tumour. Although the cancer was successfully treated, **FH** was both cognitively and physically impaired as a result. Following a lengthy period as a permanent resident at a specialist school, **FH** was supported to live in her own, adapted home with a treating clinical team and a 24-hour live-in care team, providing constant waking cover. As **FH** continued to grow in her independence, she began to express a wish to explore her sexual feelings and to have a relationship. She also expressed the wish to have a baby.

A detailed assessment was undertaken of her sexual knowledge, attitudes and beliefs, using a wide range of resources, including those available from the British Institute of Learning Disabilities, (www.bild.org.uk/product/exploring-sexual-and-social-understanding-second-edition/).

The following topics were explored with **FH** in detail, information was shared and then understanding and reasoning were assessed:

- Body parts, sexual reproduction;
- Contraception and sexual health;
- Relationships (sexual and non-sexual);
- Sexual and individual rights (to say "no"); and
- Public vs private spaces.

FH had a degree of understanding of the fact that sex between a man and woman can result in a pregnancy. She was unable to identify any negatives about having sex, such as pain or not finding it pleasurable or feeling pressured into having sex when not sure. For **FH**, sex was about having a baby. Her knowledge, despite several sessions of education (and a previous course at her residential school) was lacking. She did not understand non-heterosexual choices.

FH was unaware that consent is required throughout the sex act. She stated that, *"you've got to like the person and they have got to like you . . . you've got to trust someone"*. However, despite lengthy exploration of the concept of trust, **FH** did not actually know what "trust" means. She appeared to have some elements of concrete knowledge without a comparable level of understanding. The concept of being "safe" was explored with **FH** using Women's Health resources. It is unclear how much of this was understood.

Considerable time was spent with **FH** exploring the concepts of "yes" and "no", such as:

- *Is it ok to say no?*
- *Does no always mean no?*
- *Does yes always mean yes?*

FH was then presented with many potential scenarios for which she was asked to indicate "yes" or "no", such as "*is it ok to have sex without a condom?*" and "*is it ok to have sex when you have known each other a short time?*" (items taken from a sex and relationships course). Her responses were concrete and somewhat automatic and, although she did display some understanding of the appropriate application of "yes" and "no", this was not consistent.

FH believed that the only outcome of sex is a baby. When asked about whether or not it is a big decision to have a baby, **FH** replied that it is not, "*if you want it*".

FH was given considerable information, over several sessions, regarding different types of contraception as well as the purpose of using these. She was only able to understand very basic information. Time was spent with **FH** exploring different types of relationships, such as friend/boyfriend/husband, as well as looking at what it is "ok" to do with each in terms of appropriateness. Her thinking was concrete and muddled, despite being given the correct information.

The outcome of the assessment was to hold a Best Interests decision process at which the least restrictive and most competence-promoting assistance could be given to **FH** to acknowledge and work with her rights as a sexual being, in a safe manner. The outcome of this process was to:

- Establish opportunities for FH to meet peers so that she could develop meaningful relationships with others;
- Provide specialised education and support to FH to explore her sexual self in a safe way, including guidance for her care staff to allow her privacy within her room, whilst maintaining her safety.

The law is clear in terms of assisting a person with a disability **to access a sex worker**. In a recent case before the Court of Protection[10] (which is under Appeal at time of writing), the judge had to consider the situation of a man with capacity to consent to sex but who, at the same time, lacked capacity to manage his property and affairs or to decide upon his care and treatment.

Essentially, the man, "C", expressed the wish to have sex with a sex worker, as he realised that the prospect of having a girlfriend was limited. The Court needed to decide whether the local authority's plan to assist C in securing a sex worker constituted an offence under the Sexual Offences Act (2003).

In his judgement, Hayden J notes that,

> *The Act . . . is tailored to promoting the right to enjoy a private life, it is not structured in a way that is intended to curtail it (paragraph 90). . . . In C's case there is clear and cogent evidence that he has the capacity to engage in sexual relations and to decide to have contact with a sex worker. He understands the importance of consent both prior to and during sexual contact . . . he lacks the capacity to make the practical arrangements involved in identifying a suitable and safe sex worker and is unable to negotiate a financial transaction (paragraph 91).*

There is a resource available to assist with sourcing safe sex workers for those with disabilities (https://tlc-trust.org.uk/) which is considered in the Neuro Rehab Times (reference at end).

Key Learning Points	•	There are specific legal tests for mental capacity to enter into a pre-nuptial agreement, to marry, to engage in sex and to secure a sex worker.
	•	People with disabilities have sexual and reproductive rights (WHO, 2009).

4   Social media and internet use

Case law which specifically considers how capacity, social media and internet use should be assessed, determined that the "relevant information" which P needs to be able to understand, retain and use and weigh is as follows:[11]

> i) *Information and images (including videos) which you share on the internet or through social media could be shared more widely,*

11 [2019] EWCOP 2, 3.

including with people you don't know, without you knowing or being able to stop it;

ii) It is possible to limit the sharing of personal information or images (and videos) by using 'privacy and location settings' on some internet and social media sites;

iii) If you place material or images (including videos) on social media sites which are rude or offensive, or share those images, other people might be upset or offended;

iv) Some people you meet or communicate with ('talk to') online, who you don't otherwise know, may not be who they say they are ('they may disguise, or lie about, themselves'); someone who calls themselves a 'friend' on social media may not be friendly;

v) Some people you meet or communicate with ('talk to') on the internet or through social media, who you don't otherwise know, may pose a risk to you; they may lie to you, or exploit or take advantage of you sexually, financially, emotionally and/or physically; they may want to cause you harm;

vi) If you look at or share extremely rude or offensive images, messages or videos online you may get into trouble with the police, because you may have committed a crime.

With regard to the test above, I would like to add the following points to assist in its interpretation and application:

i) In relation to (ii) in [28] above, I do not envisage that the precise details or mechanisms of the privacy settings need to be understood but P should be capable of understanding that they exist, and be able to decide (with support) whether to apply them;

ii) In relation to (iii) and (vi) in [28] above, I use the term 'share' in this context as it is used in the 2018 Government Guidance: 'Indecent Images of Children: Guidance for Young People': that is to say, "sending on an email, offering on a file sharing platform, uploading to a site that other people have access to, and possessing with a view to distribute";

iii) In relation to (iii) and (vi) in [28] above , I have chosen the words 'rude or offensive' – as these words may be easily understood by those with learning disabilities as including not only the insulting and abusive, but also the sexually explicit, indecent or pornographic;

iv)   *In relation to (vi) in [28] above, this is not intended to represent
a statement of the criminal law, but is designed to reflect the
importance, which a capacitous person would understand, of
not searching for such material, as it may have criminal content,
and/or steering away from such material if accidentally encoun-
tered, rather than investigating further and/or disseminating
such material. Counsel in this case cited from the Government
Guidance on 'Indecent Images of Children' (see (ii) above).
Whilst the Guidance does not refer to 'looking at' illegal images
as such, a person should know that entering into this territory
is extremely risky and may easily lead a person into a form of
offending. This piece of information (in [28](vi)) is obviously
more directly relevant to general internet use rather than com-
munications by social media, but it is relevant to social media
use as well.* (paragraph 29)

*I should add that I heard argument on the issue of whether to
include in the list of relevant information that internet use may have
a psychologically harmful impact on the user. It is widely known
that internet use can be addictive; accessing legal but extreme por-
nography, radicalisation or sites displaying inter-personal violence,
for instance, could cause the viewer to develop distorted views of
healthy human relationships, and can be compulsive. Such sites
could cause the viewer distress. I take the view that many capacitous
internet users do not specifically consider this risk, or if they do, they
are indifferent to this risk. I do not therefore regard it as appropriate
to include this in the list of information relevant to the decision on
a test of capacity under section 3 MCA 2005 (paragraph 30).*

FJ was a young woman living in her own home with a
24-hour care package, who was dependent for all care needs,
and who had a developing interest in using social media. This
was an entirely age- and peer-appropriate interest, and a mental
capacity assessment was conducted on the basis that she had
begun to access unsafe sites on her smart tablet which permit-
ted others to send her (often) inappropriate messages.

FJ confirmed that she used her phone for calling and texting
her family, for gaming (on her own), for sending photographs

and e-mails and for accessing YouTube to watch videos. She used her tablet for similar functions, except phone calls. FJ kept her phone and tablet in her room overnight on some occasions and so had unsupported access to the internet. FJ was only able to identify shopping as a main use of the internet. When asked about possible other uses, and prompted to look at her tablet, she was able to identify that she also used the internet to access free gaming applications.

She was unable to identify how a game that she accessed would be safe in terms of information she might share to join a game (name, personal details, password). When asked how she would know if a game was safe, she replied, "well, it would tell you". When asked about how others might keep her safe, she replied that she would "ask for help" but gave no indication as to when (or under what circumstances) she might require assistance. FJ was unaware of who has access to her e-mail and app username and passwords and so could access her various accounts. FJ was asked about her e-mail account. She stated that her e-mails can be read by herself and her carers. She thought her dad could access her e-mails and stated that she did not mind this.

It was established that FJ used basic (and largely unsafe) passwords such as 1,2,3,4 or 1,1,1,1 to access free games. She did not consider that she needs help from her care team to choose or join a game that she likes the look of.

FJ had no understanding that any pictures or personal information that she uploaded to share with (virtual) friends might not remain private. She was asked if she posted a message or picture who might see it or how long it might remain on the internet. She had no idea. FJ was then asked what advice she would give to someone else about how to stay safe on the internet and she replied that she would tell them not to go on the internet. She stated that she had heard of the word "firewall" but did not know what it meant.

FJ was asked how she might stay safe on the internet if someone who she is in contact with sent her something inappropriate, rude or upsetting. She stated that she would "ignore the message" without understanding that she would not know until after the event. **FJ** also said that if she received an e-mail from someone or a source that she did not know, she would open it. She did not believe that there are people on the internet who pretend to be who/what they are not. However, with further discussion and exploration, **FJ** was able to see that the internet can be dangerous if people can "look at your house or know how to rob your bank".

At this point in the assessment, **FJ** started to access and play games on her tablet. As she was scrolling through her apps, it was evident that she had a large number of unopened e-mails. When asked about these, she did not know who they were from. When gaming, **FJ** did not understand that some games required a subscription before releasing a free trial of the same.

FJ was aware of some social media sites including Facebook, but not Instagram, Twitter, Whatsapp or Snapchat, for example. She was vaguely aware of Facebook, as she reported that she had previously seen a fellow pupil's Facebook pages when at school. She did say that she would want to use Facebook in her own right as a means to "chatting with" and "looking at" people. She was interested in learning more. When at her residential school, she had attended a class about use of social media and the internet but could not recall anything that she had learned.

The outcome of the assessment was that **FJ** was considered to lack capacity to make decisions around social media and internet use, and a Best Interests process was undertaken. The decision was taken, by all of those involved in supporting **FJ**, to activate safety (parental) controls on all **FJ**'s devices. This would be discussed with **FJ** in terms of keeping her safe, would be carried out by a specialist provider and would be reviewed after six months. This best interests' decision would ensure that a) active screen time could be monitored; b) restrictions could be placed on app installations to prevent inappropriate, dangerous or expensive applications; c) content filters could be activated on internet use (on browsers, e.g., SafeSearch on Chrome); and d) social relationships and interactions with strangers could be monitored.

Key Learning Points	•	Don't expect a person being assessed to "know" about social media and the negatives of internet use if these have not been explained to them.
	•	Provide as much support as possible, at the point of use, to empower the person being assessed.
	•	The Courts recognise that social media is of central importance to those with disabilities.

5 Making a Will

The common law test which states that for an individual to have testamentary capacity[12] they must be able to:

- Understand the nature of the act of Will-making;
- Understand the effects of making a Will in the form proposed;
- Understand and recollect the extent (although not necessarily the value) of the property which is being disposed of under the Will. Considerable practical difficulties can arise in relation to value where a testator's portfolio is managed by someone else and he or she does not have access to recent valuations and in those circumstances it may be necessary to apply a 'reasonableness' test; and
- Comprehend and appreciate the nature and extent of the claims upon them, both of those whom they are including in their Will and those whom they are excluding from their Will.

The tests are based mainly on understanding, that is, the ability to receive, evaluate and make a decision on information that is already known to the person making the Will. The final part of the test extends beyond mere understanding requiring other qualities such as judgement; the ability to discern, distinguish

12 *Banks v Goodfellow* (1870) LR 5 QB 549

and compare; the ability to reason; moral responsibility; memory; sentiment and affection.

The evidence and information which is available to assist in the process of this assessment may be derived from many sources, including one's own professional assessment of cognitive abilities, formal psychometric measures and evidence of those who have regular dealings with the person. The issues of influence and coercion are never far from many considerations of testamentary capacity, and there is a growing trend for family members to challenge the Will of a deceased relative on such grounds.

FL was a young lady who had sustained a traumatic brain injury and had returned to live at home. She was unable to live independently and needed considerable support due to a lack of intellectual awareness of her needs. She had recently been awarded a substantial financial settlement as a result of her personal injury claim, and, as she was estranged from several close family members, there was a concern to establish her capacity to make a Will.

Conversations were had with **FL**, her brain injury Case Manager and her mother in order to establish her level of understanding of financial matters, her knowledge of family and close friends and the impact of her brain injury in day-to-day decision-making. Reports were available from her NHS neurorehabilitation treating team, which included a Neuropsychologist. This meant that her cognitive abilities had been robustly measured recently. A previous assessment had concluded that she lacked Testamentary Capacity.

Based on her responses to a structured interview, **FL** was clear that she knew what a Will was for, when it works and what she wanted her Will to state. She was aware that she had a range of assets (property, bank accounts and investments). **FL** was not aware of the market value of her property, but this is a fact that could be established (through a professional valuation) and shared with her. She was aware that if she were to die without a Will, her wishes would not necessarily be followed. She was aware of who may have a claim on her estate after her death but had clearly reasoned arguments as to why she would not wish them to benefit directly from her Will. **FL** stated that she would need to change her planned Will were she to marry and have children, which is her wish for the future.

FL was also clear that she only wanted her mother to know the contents of her Will once it is drawn up. She did not want her family members to know the details, as she strongly wished for her personal matters to be kept confidential. She was worried that there would be arguments over her plans. She knew that she had the support of her mother and her solicitor should she wish to make any changes at any point in the future.

FL was asked about what would happen to any debts she may have on death, and she was aware that these would be paid out of her estate. She was keen to ensure that no debts were passed on to her loved ones. She was aware that her Will could be challenged but that anyone doing so would have to have a strong case and evidence to put before the Court.

Conversations with her case manager and mother corroborated her account and both considered that she had formed her opinions without external influences.

It was my opinion that **FL** did understand the nature and act of Will-making. She had clear ideas about how she wished her assets to be disposed of after her death. Her plan was clear and simple. She wished for her entire estate to be divided equally between five named beneficiaries. She did not have any specific bequests but may have benefitted from understanding what might happen if she was pre-deceased by any of the proposed beneficiaries. **FL** had a sufficient grasp of the extent of her estate even if she could not retain the exact detail or figures involved. It was relatively straightforward to provide her with this information in a form which she can refer to if needed. **FL** explained her reasoning as to why she wanted to exclude members of the wider family from her Will. She explained that she feels that the five named beneficiaries can provide, from the assets that they inherit from **FL**, for any of their family members that they wish to. Her wish was to keep her Will simple and equitable. In my opinion, on the balance of probabilities, **FL** retained Testamentary Capacity.

Rees & Ryan-Morgan (2012) describes a case in which a previously incapacitous individual was supported to make a Will.

Key Learning Points	• Even though the legal test for establishing whether or not a person has the capacity to make a Will is based on a 19th-century case, it provides a clear framework to follow.
	• Always assess the person alone to avoid the possibility that, in the future, the Will could be challenged on the basis of influence from others.

Reflections of a *professional*

Court-Appointed Deputy (Robert Thomas)

It is easy to forget as a Deputy, or as anyone tasked with making decisions for others, what an invasive role that is for the individuals about whom decisions are to be made and their families. To have what often amounts to a total stranger poking their noses into your affairs takes some getting used to and there is a need to build a bond of trust over time. This is trust that you will make appropriate decisions for the right reasons; that you will stick to your remit and not impact the family more widely, as well as trust that their personal information that you suddenly have access to will remain confidential.

A Deputy is appointed because P is deemed to lack capacity to manage their property and affairs or certain health and welfare matters. There is an innate conflict here between such a wide role and the MCA principle that capacity is issue and time specific. In relation to a financial deputy, P may lack capacity because, although they can manage smaller sums of money quite easily, they struggle with managing larger sums over longer periods of time. However, for reasons which have been addressed in the foregoing chapter, a Deputy is appointed, in theory, to do it all. Once appointed, the Deputy needs to develop an understanding of what P can do for themselves and leave them to those matters while providing a safety net for those areas where P cannot manage. The guide is to maximise their independence and their ability to make whatever decisions they can for themselves.

There are occasions when that trust can never be established, whether because of the injuries sustained, a long-standing family dynamic or the personality of the individual concerned, to name a few. This makes the decision-making process more difficult but reinforces the need for consistency in how those decisions are arrived at. You should always be willing to explain decisions and also be able to show your workings (thank you, O-Level maths!).

There will be clients who have absolutely no insight into their difficulties whatsoever and don't accept that they need help. There are families who are very private and resent outside interference. There are families who see any compensation claim as a lottery win for the family as a whole and resent someone else dictating how funds are spent. These influences make assessing capacity and any subsequent decision-making trickier than can often be assumed when considering the workings of the MCA and its guidance in a theoretical context.

When a lack of capacity is established, what may seem like an obvious decision to make can provoke enormous uproar. Other decisions, you expect to face opposition are accepted without a word being uttered. A male client in his 30s with a brain injury was found to have capacity to have sex but struggled to establish relationships because of that brain injury or to arrange an appropriate liaison in any other way. He had an itch that needed scratching, and along with the case manager and neuropsychologist, we came up with a plan that a holiday to Amsterdam would be an appropriate way forward supported by his care team. The family did not agree, and the client's father proposed chemical castration as his preferred solution to the problem. Not an option we considered for very long, and we were surprised how strongly the family objected to our initial proposal.

Providing support to P to make decisions can cause problems as well. Where sits the line between providing support and actually making the decision for them? When a decision is to be made, then helping P overcome their difficulties to make that decision themselves often means helping them understand the issue which needs to be decided by simplifying language used away from legal jargon and similar; it means taking breaks so that fatigue does not affect the retention of information or the ability to weigh up; it also means providing communication assistance so that P's decision can be passed to those who need it. However, too often the support-ive spouse or the proactive financial adviser are deemed to be the support that P needs, and so capacity is presumed because of such support and not because that support helps P make the decision. It is a fine line but one to be wary of.

Taking your time to assess capacity is important and not being rushed into decisions by P or their families. P may want to do X, and it may be all-consuming for them. They may not understand why they can't make the decision straightaway or why you won't do it for them immediately when asked. Taking the time to make a proper assessment of their capacity to make that decision is import-ant as well as buying time to consider whether, in the event of a lack of capacity, what you might do when faced with the ques-tion. Time can uncover a multitude of issues and helps avoid the ubiquitous Law of Unintended Consequences. You may also find that what was all-consuming to P at the time has now been totally forgotten as they have moved on.

Brain Injury Case Manager, Expert Witness and Occupational Therapist (Rhiannon Stokes)

As an Occupational Therapist and Case Manager, the subject of capacity is a daily occurrence for me at very different levels. It is very common for the issues around capacity to be discussed at length with the individuals themselves, families and the treating professionals. In fact, it is quite often the case that it is the Case Manager themselves that brings up the issue of needing capacity to be assessed.

I find it a very interesting area of practice within the brain injury field but also a very complex and challenging arena. I consider that as a Case Manager it is my duty to ensure that I understand the law around capacity, how it should be assessed and how I can support the individual to understand what it means to them.

It is important that any subject area is treated with the same respect and professionalism when assessment is required, and the client deserves to have every opportunity to have time spent on an assessment. There are no rules as to how long an assessment should take. I have seen it happen too many times where professionals make snap decisions on capacity, or they don't spend enough time assessing or assessing in a way that meets the individual's needs.

It is so important that Case Managers understand that they can be crucial to assisting the "capacity assessor". Of course, a case manager (with the right clinical background) can themselves assess an individual's capacity. It doesn't have to be left to a Medical Consultant or an Expert Witness within a litigation case.

It is often a misconception that it has to be a Neuropsychologist or Neuropsychiatrist that carries out capacity assessments.

In my experience as a Case Manager, it is imperative that when supporting a capacity assessment, I support the client to understand what area of capacity is being assessed. Communication is the key here and there are times when we have to call on other health professionals to also provide help.

For example, I have had to ask for a Speech and Language Therapist to meet with me and the client to use picture cards to help the client understand what is being discussed. Quite often pictures and diagrams can assist spoken language. If they work with a Speech and Language Therapist, then that professional will know more about the best way to communicate; using the team around you is so helpful.

Repetition is also incredibly beneficial, as individuals with a brain injury can take longer to process information or may well have memory difficulties. Going back over the details of the pre-assessment or the assessment is vital. I have recorded/videoed sessions previously (with consent) and found that playing them back can assist the client to process information. They need every opportunity to be able to take on board the information and issues that are being discussed.

I have found that being interviewed by a capacity assessor or providing a detailed report can assist the assessments. Case Managers have access to the evidence on the ground. We read the support worker notes daily, we know how the families are managing or not managing. We often have a good understanding of the way the individual lived their life prior to a brain injury or what values and standards were held in their life.

Case Managers are key to monitoring and managing the individual's rehabilitation and/or support. It might be that a individuals capacity changes or fluctuates, and if it does, then this must be documented and communicated to the right professionals. The management of finances is a good example. After a brain injury, an individual has a lot to cope with. They might have significant cognitive and psychological difficulties that impact their ability to manage money. At that point in time, they may need support to manage funds and daily administration. An assessment may deem them not to have capacity. However, as time goes on, they might develop coping strategies and support networks that will allow their capacity to change.

Professionals and families should not make assumptions that if an individual has a brain injury, then they can't possibly have capacity or won't ever have capacity again. This is just not the case.

Resources and weblinks

https://assets.publishing.service.gov.uk/government/uploads/system/uploads/attachment_data/file/921428/Mental-capacity-act-code-of-practice.pdf

Rees, S. J. & Ryan-Morgan, T. (2012) An exercise for maximising capacity in decision making. *Journal of Social Care and Neurodisability*, *3* (2), pp. 69–76.

Sex and Rehab. (2019) *Neuro Rehab Times*, Issue 9, Q1, pp. 38–43.

WHO. (2009) www.who.int/reproductivehealth/publications/general/9789241598682/en/

www.bild.org.uk/product/exploring-sexual-and-social-understanding-second-edition/

Index

13; repetition of information 137;
support to assessees 11, 13
metabolic disorders 34–36
Montreal Cognitive Assessment
(MOCA) 27
Moore, S. 87
Mostyn, Justice 119
Multiple Errands Task 59, 90–92
Munby, Justice 118

neglect *see* wilful mistreatment and
neglect
Newton, Justice 12
NICE 3, 5, 9, 10, 11, 86

one-off decisions 12
one-to-one care 55
oral evidence in Court of Protection
96–99
Organic Personality Disorder (OPD)
89–90, 116

pain 36
Parker, Justice 88
performative decisions *see* repeated
decisions
Prader Willi Syndrome 34
pre-nuptial agreement 119–120
property and affairs 14–16, 89–90,
92, 102, 113–118, 138

real-world behaviours, observation
of 29, 86, 90–91
recall of information 4, 45

Rees, S. J. 134
reflective system 25–26, 35
Relevant Person's Representative
(RPR) 47, 49, 50, 53
repeated decisions 12
research, consent to participate 7
residence 80, 107, 112
restraints 71, 84
Ruck-Keene, A. 4, 10, 11, 12, 13,
19, 88, 96, 101
Ryan-Morgan, T. 7, 134

sexual activity 5–6, 122–125
sex workers, accessing
125–126
social media *see* internet use and
social media
Standard Authorisation
52–53
strategy application disorder 34
substance misuse 37–39

threshold of understanding
4, 10
Tower Test 28

undue influence 40–41
Urgent Authorisation 52–53

wilful mistreatment and neglect
7, 76
Will, making 6, 7, 101, 131–134
Wisconsin Card Sort 28
Wood, R. L. 29

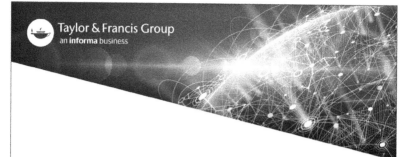